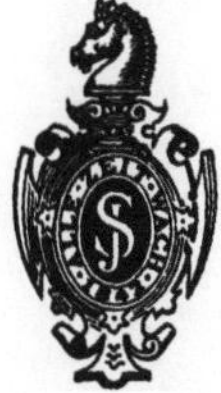

Recent Results in Cancer Research

Fortschritte der Krebsforschung

Progrès dans les recherches sur le cancer

27

Edited by

*V. G. Allfrey, New York · M. Allgöwer, Basel · K. H. Bauer, Heidelberg
I. Berenblum, Rehovoth · F. Bergel, Jersey · J. Bernard, Paris · W. Bernhard, Villejuif · N. N. Blokhin, Moskva · H. E. Bock, Tübingen · P. Bucalossi, Milano · A. V. Chaklin, Moskva · M. Chorazy, Gliwice · G. J. Cunningham, Richmond · W. Dameshek †, Boston · M. Dargent, Lyon · G. Della Porta, Milano · P. Denoix, Villejuif · R. Dulbecco, La Jolla · H. Eagle, New York
R. Eker, Oslo · P. Grabar, Paris · H. Hamperl, Bonn · R. J. C. Harris, London
E. Hecker, Heidelberg · R. Herbeuval, Nancy · J. Higginson, Lyon
W. C. Hueper, Fort Myers · H. Isliker, Lausanne · D. A. Karnofsky †, New York · J. Kieler, København · G. Klein, Stockholm · H. Koprowski, Philadelphia · L. G. Koss, New York · G. Martz, Zürich · G. Mathé, Villejuif
O. Mühlbock, Amsterdam · W. Nakahara, Tokyo · V. R. Potter, Madison
A. B. Sabin, Rehovoth · L. Sachs, Rehovoth · E. A. Saxén, Helsinki
W. Szybalski, Madison · H. Tagnon, Bruxelles · R. M. Taylor, Toronto
A. Tissières, Genève · E. Uehlinger, Zürich · R. W. Wissler, Chicago
T. Yoshida, Tokyo*

Editor in chief

P. Rentchnick, Genève

Springer-Verlag Berlin · Heidelberg · New York 1970

Janusz Szymendera

Bone Mineral Metabolism
in Cancer

With 43 Figures

Springer-Verlag Berlin · Heidelberg · New York 1970

Janusz Szymendera, M. D., Research Assistant in Nuclear Medicine,
Department of Isotopes, Institute of Oncology, Warsaw 22, Poland

Sponsored by the Swiss League against Cancer

ISBN-13: 978-3-642-99980-2   e-ISBN-13: 978-3-642-99978-9
DOI: 10.1007/978-3-642-99978-9

Introduction

The introduction of new methods for studying the plasma state, renal handling, and kinetics of calcium and inorganic phosphate has rendered possible a more efficient and appropriate approach to the problems of bone-tissue metabolism and more adequate investigation of the pathogenesis of its miscellaneous abnormalities. Used to study the metabolism of bone mineral in osteoporosis, hypo- and hyperparathyroidism, and other metabolic bone diseases, the new methods have given much valuable information. In malignancy they also promise to supplement the scantiness of the existing information better than the routine examination procedures, yet they have been used far more rarely in this field.

The material presented in this work represents an attempt to marshal the facts and to answer, by the aid of recent techniques, some still open problems of bone-mineral metabolism in patients with cancer. Since the new techniques involve an entirely new approach, the first two chapters are devoted to it and details of these techniques are presented in the third chapter.

I realize the shortcomings of this work, but the never-ending and continuously increasing search for new discoveries makes some data obsolete at the moment of their presentation. Nevertheless, I hope that this work will give some information which will be useful in interpreting disturbances of bone-tissue metabolism in patients, both without any evidence of bone secondaries, and with widespread osseous metastases.

Warsaw, February 1970   Janusz Szymendera

Foreword

This study was carried out over the last eight years at the Department of Isotopes, Institute of Oncology, Warsaw. I wish to express my sincere gratitude to my chief, Professor WŁADYSŁAW K. JASIŃSKI, M. D., for his suggestion about the study, for his interest in it, and for his kindness in placing the facilities of the Department at my disposal.

I am greatly indebted to my colleagues and friends, JERZY TOŁWIŃSKI, Ph. D., for his valuable suggestions and help in the mathematical treatment and presentation of the results, and CZESŁAW SMARSZ, Ph. D., for kind supply and informations on the use of ultrafiltration devices, and for helpful discussions during the present work.

I am grateful to MAURICE E. SHILS, M. D., Sc. D., Associate Member of the Sloan-Kettering Institute for Cancer Research, for advice on metabolic balance investigations and for kindly supplying a brillant blue dye.

I owe my sincerest thanks to the members of the metabolic team, STEFAN MADA-JEWICZ, M. B., JANUSZ NOWOSIELSKI, M. Sc., Mrs. CHRISTINA ROGALSKA, technical assistant, and Mrs. SOPHIE MOZER, dietitian, for their collaboration and technical assistance, without which the work would have been impossible.

I am also greatly indebted to Assistant Professor ADAM MICHAŁOWSKI, M. D., who helped me in preparing the English manuscript.

This study was supported by grants from the International Atomic Energy Agency, the Polish Academy of Sciences and the Medical Academy of Warsaw.

Contents

Chapter 1

General Outlines of Bone Tissue Metabolism

Bones are organized on two levels: as organs and as a tissue. As organs, they are particular elements of the skeleton adapted to withstand stresses; as a tissue, they form a highly specialized connective tissue composed of cells embedded in an interstitial substance, which includes the organic framework or matrix and the mineral. A brief account of what is known about the molecular structure and metabolism of the major parts of bone—cells, organic matrix and inorganic salts—seems advisable.

1. Structure and Function of Bone Cells

Bone cells are organized in three compartments: a proliferating, a functional, and a final-stage compartment (OWEN, 1963). The first compartment cells, the pre-osteoblasts, are reproducing themselves, and the second compartment cells may be either osteoblasts or osteoclasts. The final-stage cell of an osteoblast is the osteocyte (OWEN, 1963).

Osteoblasts and osteocytes have much the same fine structure and reveal the cytoplasmatic features of intense metabolic activity: they control the metabolism of collagen, proteoglycans and glycoproteins, as well as the mineral elements of bone tissue (BAUD, 1966). Osteoclasts, giant cells with a variable number of nuclei, produce organic acids, the agents of the solubilization of bone mineral, as well as acid hydrolases—the enzymes that digest organic matrix (VAES, 1966). There is good evidence to suggest that bone cells of all functional states stem from the preosteoblast (OWEN, 1963).

The differences in structure and metabolic activities of bone cells are associated with their specific function: osteoblasts with formation, osteocytes with maintenance, and osteoclasts with resorption of bone (BAUER et al., 1961).

2. Structure and Function of Bone Matrix

The interstitial organic substance or matrix consists of two major components: collagen and ground substance.

2.1. Collagen

Composition and Structure of Collagen

The collagenous framework of the bone tissue is composed of typical fibres having characteristic low-angle X-ray diffraction patterns and banded patterns in the electron microscope with a periodicity of 64—70 nm (RAMACHANDRAN, 1963). Each collagen fibre is composed of basic tropocollagen molecules having a molecular weight of 300,000 (BORNSTEIN and PIEZ, 1964), a length of 300 nm, and a diameter of 1.5—1.6 nm in the wet state (BEAR, 1952).

Tropocollagen is composed of three polypeptide alpha chains having the same molecular weight of about 100,000. The alpha 2 chain differs in its amino acid composition and chromatographic behaviour from the two alpha 1 chains (BORNSTEIN and PIEZ, 1964). The amino acid composition of alpha 1 and alpha 2 chains of human skin collagen—there are about 1,100 amino acid residues in each chain—is shown in Fig. 1.

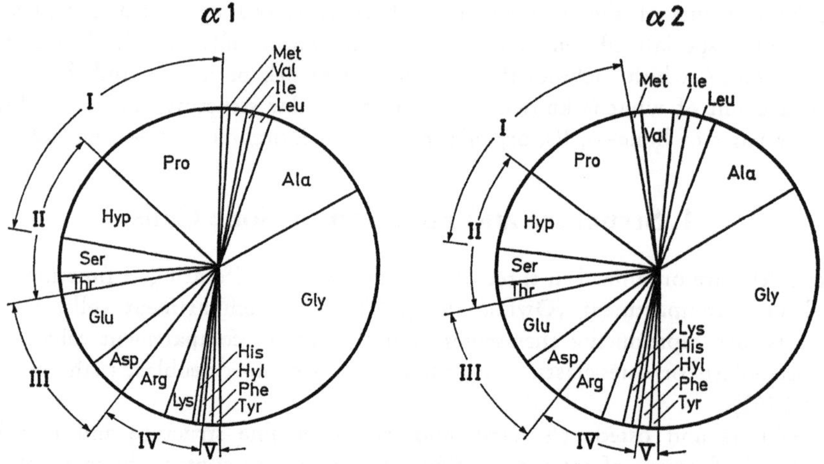

Fig. 1. A comparison of the amino acid composition of alpha chains from human skin collagen. The values used for constructing this diagram were taken from BORNSTEIN and PIEZ (1964). 1° = 2.78 amino acid residues per 1000 total residues; I = Imino acids; II = Hydroxy amino acids; III = Acidic amino acids; IV = Basic amino acids; V = Aromatic amino acids

Significant differences may be found in the contents of proline, hydroxyproline, alanine, lysine and glutamic acid (more in alpha 1 chain) and hydroxylysine, histidine, leucine, isoleucine, valine and tyrosine (more in alpha 2 chain) in comparing both chains (BORNSTEIN and PIEZ, 1964). The findings that collagen from codfish skin contains three different, chromatographically separable alpha chains (PIEZ, 1964), that the fragments produced by cleavage of the methionyl bonds in the alpha 1 chains demonstrate large variations in their amino acid composition (BORNSTEIN and PIEZ, 1965), and that the primary structure of collagen is heterogeneous as a consequence of the incomplete hydroxylation of individual prolyl residues in collagen (BORNSTEIN, 1967)—all indicate that alpha 1 chains are not identical. Moreover, the finding of large variations in amino acid composition in the fragments produced by cleavage of the methionyl bonds indicates that the amino acid sequence of each of the alpha chains is unique throughout its length (BORNSTEIN and PIEZ, 1965). It contradicts the model of collagen structure proposed by PETRUSKA and HODGE (1964) based on identical intrachain subunits.

The alpha chains of the tropocollagen molecule have a discernible recurrence of certain similar sequences of amino acids. These sequences are found in the crystalline or non-polar regions. The non-polar regions alternate with a large polypeptide run, the amorphous or polar region. The non-polar regions which form 50—60 per cent of an alpha chain are visualized as interbands in the electron micrographs, while the alternating polar regions are visualized as bands (SEIFTER et al., 1965). The attack of bacterial collagenase on non-polar sequences gives 5—6 dialysable tripeptides Gly-Pro-R, in which R represents any amino acid residue (GRASSMANN et al., 1963). The polar segments give rise to non-dialysable peptides containing from 11 to 15 residues, in which every third one is the glycyl residue, and among the other residues there are those from acidic and basic amino acids (FRANZBLAU et al., 1964). The model of the alpha chain of tropocollagen is as follows:

$$\text{-(Gly-Pro-R)}_n\text{-polar region-(Gly-Pro-R)}_n\text{-polar region-}$$
$$\text{-(Gly-Pro-R)}_n\text{-polar region-(Gly-Pro-R)}_n\text{-}$$

The peptides released by the action of pronase or pepsin, mainly from the C-terminal end of the alpha chains—to which the name telopeptides has been given—have a composition unlike that of collagen, since glycine occurs in every second position and is sandwiched between two polar amino acids, such as aspartic acid, glutamic acid, lysine, arginine and serine (ROSMUS et al., 1967; DEYL et al., 1967).

The alpha chains aggregate to form beta components, which can be of two types if the cross-link is intramolecular: beta-11 dimer of two alpha 1 chains (or, more properly, of one alpha 1 and one alpha 3 chain), and beta-12 dimer of alpha 1 and alpha 2 chain. The beta components aggregate further with one additional alpha chain to form a gamma component, which is a gamma-112 triplet (or, more properly, a gamma-123 triplet) of two alpha 1-chains and one alpha 2-chain, if the cross-linkages are intramolecular (BORNSTEIN and PIEZ, 1964; STEVEN, 1966; MILLER et al., 1967). The cross-linkages in beta and gamma components, as well as the polymerized collagen, are probably situated in the region of the telopeptides (WORRALL and STEVEN, 1966). Mature collagens contain several different types of cross-linkage with different lability towards the attack of cleaving substances (STEVEN, 1966). The quantitative differences between hard and soft tissue collagens lie in the direction of a greater extent of cross-linkages in bone collagen than in the soft tissue collagens (MILLER et al., 1967).

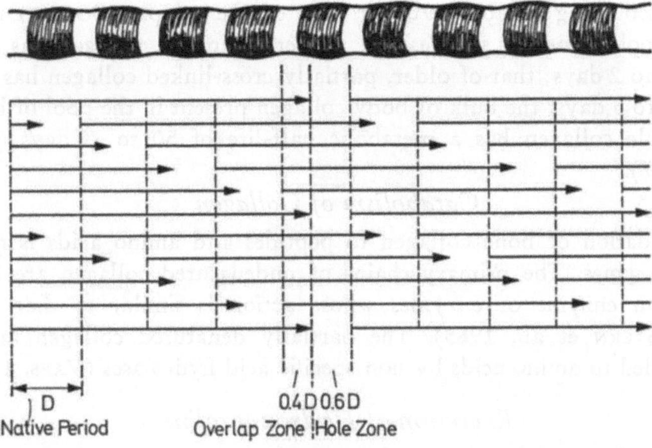

Fig. 2. A diagrammatic representation of the quarter-stagger arrangement of tropocollagen molecules in the fibril of native collagen, as advocated by PETRUSKA and HODGE

The three helically coiled alpha chains form the tropocollagen molecule (RAMA-CHANDRAN, 1963). The tropocollagen molecules are packed in the staggered array represented in Fig. 2. The quarter-stagger arrangement results in formation of fibrils of period D, with each period comprising an overlap zone of 0.4 D and a hole zone of 0.6 D (PETRUSKA and HODGE, 1964; SMITH, 1968).

Collagen Synthesis and Maturation

The synthesis of bone collagen takes place in microsomes of osteoblasts and osteo-cytes; on polysomes, that is, on polyribosomal clusters containing some scores of 70S ribosomes assembled on the messenger-RNA coded for the particular protein (MANNER et al., 1967). The amino acids are initially activated by ATP to form high-energy complexes of amino acid and AMP. The activated amino acids are then transferred to transfer-RNA. These amino acyl t-RNA compounds function as the immediate pre-cursors and are incorporated into polypeptide chain growing on the ribosomal template (WATSON, 1963). The synthesized polypeptide chains, called protocollagen, are rich in proline and lysine and free from their hydroxyderivatives. The hydroxy-lation of most of the appropriate proline residues in the polypeptide precursors of collagen occurs after completed protocollagen chains are released from ribosomal complexes (ROSENBLOOM et al., 1967; BHATNAGAR et al., 1967). The hydroxylation is effected by protocollagen hydroxylase which requires oxygen, ferrous iron, alpha-ketoglutarate and ascorbate (KIVIRIKKO and PROCKOP, 1967). The time taken to synthesize a complete protocollagen polypeptide chain is about 1 minute, but over 10 minutes are required to obtain maximal hydroxylation of the newly-synthesized polypeptide (ROSENBLOOM et al., 1967). As a result of the protocollagen hydroxyla-tion, alpha chains are built up, which are then extruded into the extracellular matrix and with time become intra- and inter-molecular cross-linked (STERN et al., 1965).

There is a close relationship between the intra- and inter-molecular cross-linking of collagens and their solubility. In neutral salt-extracted collagen, the alpha chains predominate, accounting for 70 per cent of the sample. In acid-extracted collagen there are larger amounts of beta components, accounting for 60—70 per cent of the sample. The guanidine-extracted collagen contains beta components and higher aggregates, accounting for over 70 per cent of the sample (BORNSTEIN and PIEZ, 1964). The pool of newly synthesized, not cross-linked, collagen has a metabolic half-life of 1 to 2 days; that of older, partially cross-linked collagen has a metabolic half-life of 2 to 3 days; the bulk of body collagen present in the pool of highly cross-linked insoluble collagen has a metabolic half-life of 50 to 70 days (AVIOLI and PROCKOP, 1967).

Catabolism of Collagen

The degradation of bone collagen to peptides and amino acids is mediated by proteolytic enzymes. The primary chains of undenatured collagen are degraded to peptides by an enzyme or enzymes whose action is similar to that of bacterial collagenase (STERN et al., 1965). The partially denatured collagen molecules are further degraded to amino acids by non-specific acid hydrolases (VAES, 1966).

Excretion of Hydroxyproline

Hydroxyproline can be used to follow changes in the metabolism of collagen, since essentially all is found in collagen, except for a small amount in elastine (NEU-

MAN and LOGAN, 1950), and since the only reaction by which it can be synthesized is the hydroxylation of proline after completed protocollagen chain is released from ribosomal complexes (ROSENBLOOM et al., 1967; BHATNAGAR et al., 1967).

Patients on a hydroxyproline-free diet excrete in the urine significant amounts of this imino acid originating from the degradation of collagen (PROCKOP, 1964). A comparison of the specific activity of hydroxyproline-^{14}C in the urine with that in pools of soluble and insoluble collagen suggests that about a third of the urinary hydroxyproline originates from the degradation of newly synthesized collagen, while the remainder comes from the degradation of less soluble and insoluble collagens (AVIOLI and PROCKOP, 1967). The isotopic experiments indicate that about 5 to 10 per cent of the hydroxyproline released by the degradation is excreted in the urine (PROCKOP, 1964; PROCKOP and KIVIRIKKO, 1967), and the rest is oxidized by hydroxyproline oxidase to Δ'-pyrroline-3-hydroxy-5-carboxylate and ultimately to carbon dioxide and urea (EFRON et al., 1968).

2.2. Ground Substance

Composition and Structure of Ground Substance

The ground substance, in which the cells and collagen are embedded, consists of proteoglycans and glycoproteins. The saccharide components of proteoglycans are galactosaminoglycans and glucosaminoglycans, and those of glycoproteins—sialic acid, hexosamine, hexose and pentose (BARRETT, 1968). The proteins of ground substance are of fibrous and globular nature (FITTON JACKSON, 1965).

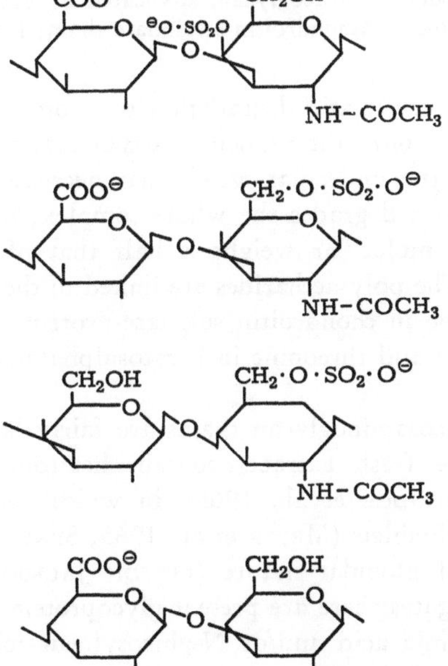

Fig. 3. Structures of repeating disaccharide units of glycosaminoglycans. C-4-S = Chondroitin 4-sulphate; C-6-S = Chondroitin 6-sulphate; KS = Keratosulphate; Hyal = Hyaluronate

Galactosaminoglycans are polymer molecules consisting of repeating units of either chondroitin 4-sulphate (C-4-S) or chondroitin 6-sulphate (C-6-S). Both units contain beta-glucuronic acid and N-acetylgalactosamine with ester sulphates at C_4 (C-4-S) or at C_6 (C-6-S) (DAVIDSON and SMALL, 1963). Glucosaminoglycans are polymer molecules consisting of repeating units of keratosulphate (KS) containing galactose and N-acetylglucosamine with ester sulphate at C_6 (DAVIDSON and SMALL, 1963). Keratosulphate exhibits a high degree of heterogeneity; it varies in galactose content alternating with L-fucose or 6-desoxy-L-galactose (SENO et al., 1965). The polymer molecules consist of a linear succession of some scores of repeating units. A polymer containing two ore more ester sulphates in some repeating units is designated as sulphated glycosaminoglycan. Another polymer molecule, hyaluronic acid (HYAL), consists of repeating units containing beta-glucuronic acid and N-acetylglucosamine (BARRETT, 1968). Structures of repeating units are presented in Fig. 3.

The proteoglycan complexes consist of glycosaminoglycans covalently linked to a species-specific protein core (FITTON JACKSON, 1965), in all likelihood, in a comb-like fashion (MATHEWS and LOSAITYTE, 1958), as shown in Fig. 4.

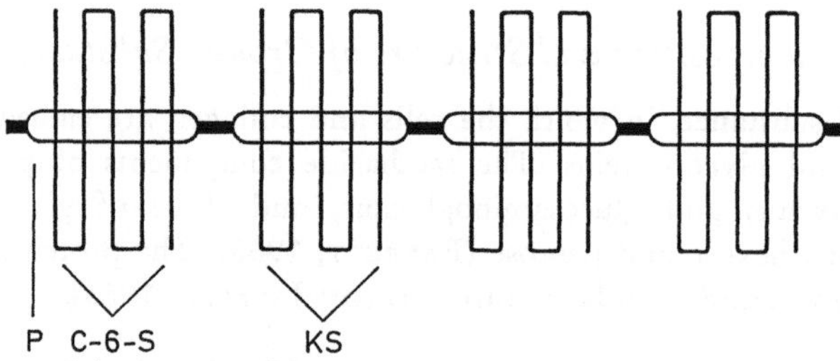

Fig. 4. Comb-like model of proteoglycan, advocated by MATHEWS and LOSAITYTE. P = Protein core; C-6-S = Chondroitin 6-sulphate chain; KS = Keratosulphate chain

The kinetics of enzymatic degradation of proteoglycans supports this structure. Hyaluronidase splits only the reducing saccharides; by the time 50 per cent of the bonds are broken, the molecular weight has decreased to only 75 per cent of the initial weight. Papain degrades the whole complex; by the time 10 per cent of the bonds are broken, molecular weight is half that of the initial value (CESSI and BERNARDI, 1965). The polysaccharides are linked to the protein backbone via 0-glycoside bonds: to serine in chondroitin sulphate-protein complexes (RODÉN and SMITH, 1966), and to serine and threonine in keratosulphate-protein complexes (SENO et al., 1965).

Though the glycosaminoglycan chains are fairly homogeneous in their degree of polymerization, the fresh extracts contain heterodisperse particles in the range 1—5 million (PARTRIDGE et al., 1965), in which keratosulphates and chondroitin sulphates occur as doublets (MEYER et al., 1965; SENO et al., 1965) joined by another protein, possibly of globular nature (FITTON JACKSON, 1965). In addition to the proteoglycan aggregates there are present glycoproteins, mainly with sialic acid, that is, N-acetylneuraminic acid and/or N-glucosylneuraminic acid, presented in Fig. 5 (PARTRIDGE et al., 1965; FERRI, 1959). Since neuraminidase liberates most of the sialic acid residues, it is presumed that sialate occupies a terminal position in the molecule (FERRI, 1959).

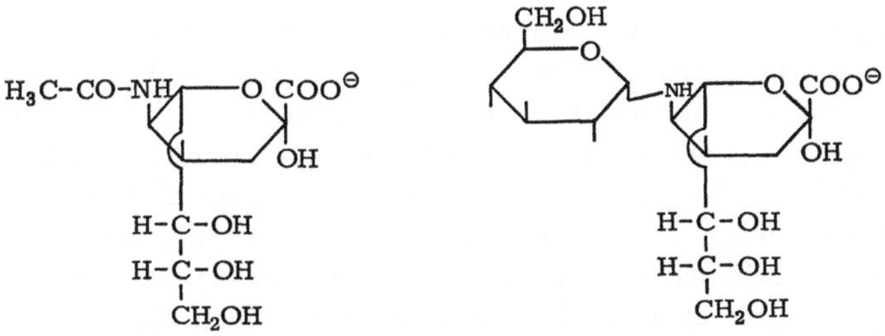

Fig. 5. Structure of sialates: N-acetylneuraminate (left) and N-glucosylneuraminate (right)

Synthesis of Proteoglycans and Glycoproteins

The synthesis of proteoglycans and glycoproteins occurs in microsomes of the same cells as collagen, that is, osteoblasts and osteocytes (BHATNAGAR and PROCKOP, 1966). Nevertheless, the pathways for the synthesis of proteoglycans and collagen are independent of each other. The polypeptide chains forming the backbone of proteoglycans are synthesized on the ribosomal template. After the completed polypeptide chains are released from the ribosomal complexes, a molecule of xylose is incorporated and followed by two molecules of galactose and some scores of glycosaminoglycan units (BARRETT, 1968). The nucleotides, uridine diphosphate derivatives of xylose, hexoses, hexosamines, and uronic acids, are the requisites for the synthesis of glycosaminoglycans (DORFMAN, 1965). The stoichiometric amounts of hexose or uronic acid and N-acetylhexosamine are synthesized alternately by a specific synthetase in the presence of Mg^{2+} (DORFMAN, 1965). Addition of sulphate to form the ester sulphate groups of polysaccharide is the terminal step in the biosynthesis of proteoglycans. It is possible that some sulphation takes place at the same time as polymerization, while additional sulphation continues after the formation of glycosaminoglycan chain (SILBERT, 1967). Sulphation occurs via transfer of sulphate from 3'-phosphoadenylylsulphate by the action of sulphotransferase (D'ABRAMO and LIPMANN, 1957). The rate-limiting step for proteoglycan synthesis is the synthesis of the peptide backbone (ADAMSON and ANAST, 1966). Sialic acid is being transferred to a polypeptide in the last step in the biosynthesis of glycoproteins (HASSID, 1967).

In the human foetus there are equal amounts of chondroitin 4-sulphate and chondroitin 6-sulphate, and insignificant amounts of keratosulphate. During the skeleton maturation, chondroitin 4-sulphate is progressively replaced by chondroitin 6-sulphate with a continuous increase in the keratosulphate. The overall content of proteoglycans falls to half the initial value (DAVIDSON and SMALL, 1963; SENO et al., 1965).

Catabolism of Proteoglycans and Glycoproteins

The time-dependent changes in the content of proteoglycans are due to their half-lives. Chondroitin sulphates exhibit short half-lives, whereas keratosulphate appears to be extremely inert following its synthesis and has a half-life resembling that of mature collagen (DAVIDSON and SMALL, 1963).

The catabolism of sulphated glycosaminoglycans depends on the desulphation processes, followed by the degradation of the desulphated polymer (LLOYD et al., 1965). DANISHEFSKY and EIBER (1959) reported the appearance in urine in very high amounts of only inorganic radiosulphate following the administration of ^{35}S-heparin, while the saccharide molecule of heparin was found not to be hydrolysed in the blood. Owing to this pathway of catabolism, normal urin contains a small amount of glycosaminoglycans, except in some mucopolysaccharidoses (KAPLAN et al., 1968). The incorporation of sulphate at the terminal point of synthesis of proteoglycans, and its cleavage in the catabolism process, both point to radiosulphate as a particularly suitable indicator for studying the ground substance metabolism.

Extensive catabolism is limited to highly polymerized substances, while low-molecular-weight carbohydrates are mainly excreted in the urine. Following the injection of ^{35}S-sulphate esters of hexoses and hexosamines, the excretion of radioactivity was 95 per cent in 48 hours, comprising over 80 per cent of unchanged esters (LLOYD et al., 1965).

3. Bone Mineral

The inorganic portion of bone contains two major mineral phases: amorphous or non-crystalline calcium phosphate, and crystalline bone apatite (TERMINE and POSNER, 1966; TERMINE and POSNER, 1967).

Chemistry and Structure of Bone Mineral

In the amorphous calcium phosphate the X-ray diffraction, infrared spectroscopy, and electron spin resonance spectroscopy, all demonstrated a lack of periodic order (TERMINE and POSNER, 1966; TERMINE and POSNER, 1967). The size and shape of this solid, exhibiting the molar Ca/P ratio of about 1.33, is not elucidated. It is possible that amorphous calcium phosphate exists both as very small particles and as their larger aggregates, since the well-known synthetic solid exhibits also a large particle-size range with an average surface area of 60 m²/g; the line of argument being that, if the amorphous calcium phosphate of bone were present as small particles only, the average surface area of bone mineral would be larger (TERMINE and POSNER, 1967). The amorphous bone mineral is metastable with respect to bone apatite.

The crystalline bone apatite fraction has an approximate composition given by the general formula $Ca_{10-x}H_{2x}(PO_4)_6(OH)_2$, where $x = 0$, 1 and 2 (GLIMCHER, 1960), and a crystal lattice near to that of hydroxyapatite given by the formula $Ca_{10}(PO_4)_6(OH)_2$ (POSNER, 1960). Both formulae represent the unit cell content, that is, the fundamental chemical repeating unit in the three-dimensional symmetry pattern of the crystal. The arrangement of the atoms in the unit cell of hydroxyapatite is shown in Fig. 6. It is seen that each phosphorus atom is surrounded by four equidistant oxygen atoms forming a tetrahedral PO_4^{3-} group, and each hydroxyl ion is surrounded by six calcium ions (POSNER, 1960). The unit cell dimensions are of $a = b = 0.94$ nm and $c = 0.69$ nm, and the bone apatite crystals form platelets with the long dimension above 20 nm, and with a width of about 2—5 nm (ENGSTRÖM, 1960). The long axis of the crystal lies parallel with the fibre axis of the collagen. Synthetic apatites comparable to cortical bone apatite in average crystal size have the surface area, as determined by low-angle X-ray scattering technique, of the order of 400 m²/g (TERMINE and POSNER, 1967).

The bone apatite crystals are calcium-deficient apatites, due to defects in the crystalline lattice and isomorphous substitutions, that is, replacement of some ions by others in the crystal without disrupting the general symmetry in both the synthetic crystals and the minerals. The calcium ion may be replaced by strontium, barium,

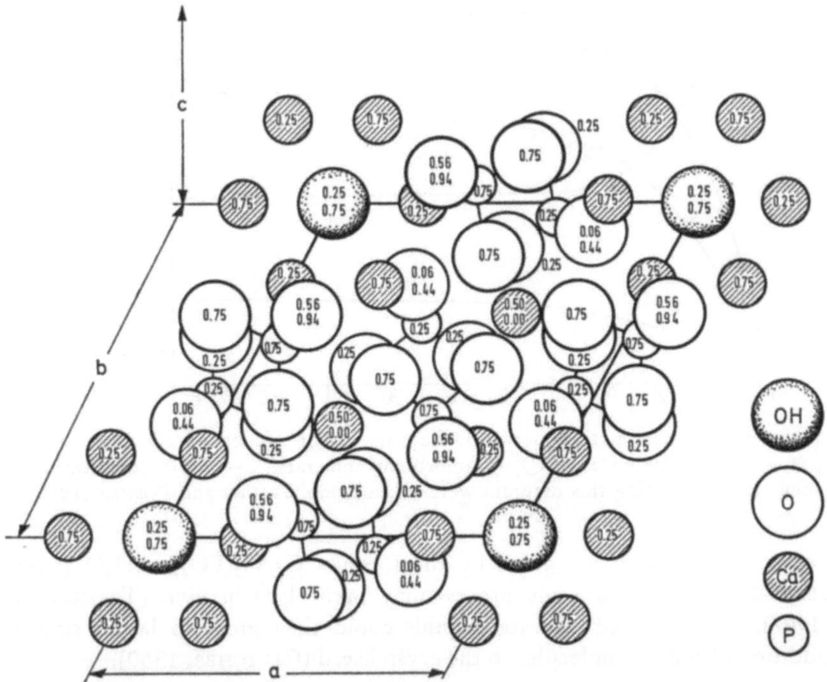

Fig. 6. The structure of the unit cell of hydroxypatite. The values within the atoms represent the height in the c-axis direction in fractions of this axis. (From POSNER, 1960)

lead, magnesium, sodium and potassium; and the hydroxyl ion by fluoride and chloride (POSNER, 1960).

The remaining ions, such as citrate and carbonate, are probably not structural constituents of bone apatites, but are adsorbed to either of major bone solids or admixed as separate phases (POSNER, 1960). Recently PELLEGRINO and BILTZ (1968) provided evidence that at least some of the calcium carbonate constitutes an integral component of bone crystal, given by the formula $Ca_9(PO_4)_6 \cdot CaCO_3$, and that only an excess of carbonate exists in a separate phase as calcium carbonate.

Amorphous/Crystalline Mineral Composition

Young bone tissue was found to be richer in amorphous mineral than in crystalline apatite. With increasing age, this relationship is gradually reversed until, at maturity, there is a constant level of both phases of mineral, and mature bone contains more crystalline apatite than amorphous solid, as seen in Fig. 7 (TERMINE and POSNER, 1966; TERMINE and POSNER, 1967).

Since the amorphous calcium phosphate appears to predominate over crystalline apatite in the early stages of bone formation, this solid is most likely the first mineral deposited during new bone formation (TERMINE et al., 1967). Synthetic, metastable amorphous calcium phosphate is also the first mineral to be converted into crystalline apatite (LERCH and VUILLEUMIER, 1966). Amorphous calcium phosphate, both synthetic (EANES and POSNER, 1965) and skeletal (TERMINE and POSNER, 1967), converts spontaneously in aqueous media into crystalline apatite via dissolution and reprecipi-

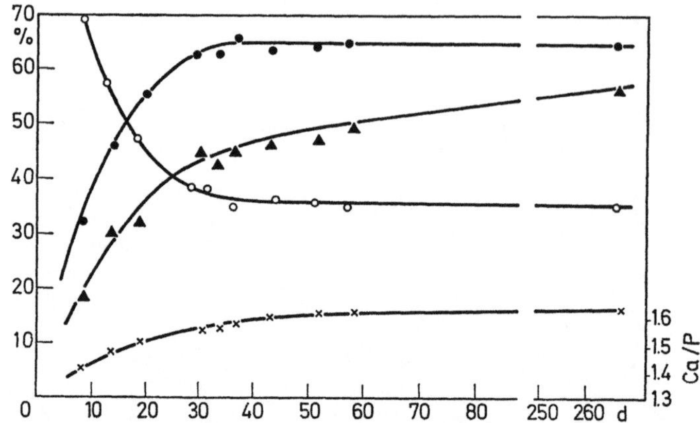

Fig. 7. Age-dependent interrelation between the two major phases of rat bone mineral. ▲ — Ash; ● — Crystalline mineral; ○ — Amorphous mineral; ✕ — Ca/P molar ratio. The values used for constructing this diagram were taken from TERMINE and POSNER (1966)

tation as octacalcium phosphate given by the formula $Ca_8H_2(PO_4)_6 \cdot xH_2O$ (LERCH and VUILLEUMIER, 1966). The same process may take place in vivo (TERMINE and POSNER, 1967). Once formed, apatite crystals could then grow to larger sizes by stepwise addition of ions or molecules to the crystal seed (GLIMCHER, 1960).

Properties of Bone Mineral

Both the amorphous calcium phosphate and crystalline apatite are strongly hydrated; the volume of hydration shell is several times greater than that of mineral. This shell contains ions in equilibrium with both the extracellular fluid and the crystal surface (McLEAN and BUDY, 1964).

The structure of apatite, its high degree of hydration, and a variable degree of charge asymmetry due to the one-to-one isomorphous replacements of divalent calcium of the crystal surface with univalent cations, all suggest this solid to be chemically reactive (PAK and BARTTER, 1967 a, b). The physico-chemical mechanism of interaction between the bone mineral and the ions of the bathing extracellular. fluid represents the exchange processes, involving three compartments in the crystal phase: hydration shell, crystal surface, and crystal interior. The half-times of calcium exchange with the hydration shell are less than 1 hour, those with the crystal surface—less than 10 hours, and those with the crystal interior—less than 65 hours (PAK and BARTTER, 1967 a, b).

Amorphous calcium phosphate of bone is even more reactive chemically than bone apatite, since amorphous solids are always at at higher energy state than are crystalline solids of similar composition (PRINS, 1965). The kinetics of calcium exchange with bone amorphous solid is not known. Since bone contains both solids, the net properties of bone mineral are dependent on the ratio of the components (TERMINE and POSNER, 1967).

Both the ionic interaction of calcium with bone mineral and the conversion of amorphous calcium phosphate into crystalline apatite via dissolution and reprecipitation might possibly be of significance in calcium homeostasis.

Mineralization of Bone

Extracellular fluid is the main source of ions for calcification and its ion product $[Ca^{2+}] \cdot [PO_4^{3-}]$ is about 1.3 $[mM]^2$. In straight solutions, resembling the extracellular fluid in ionic strength of 0.16 and pH of 7.4, the minimum ion product required to initiate hydroxyapatite crystals is of 4 $[mM]^2$; the addition of nucleating collagen lowers it to a value similar to that of extracellular fluid (FLEISCH and NEUMAN, 1961). The property of inducing formation of appropriate crystals and controlling their further growth is exihibited by the native type collagen only (GLIMCHER, 1960; FLEISCH and NEUMAN, 1961).

The mechanism of heterogeneous nucleation has not been fully elucidated. It is presumed that the nucleation centres bind orthophosphate ion which acts as a seed crystal. Until quite recently it was presumed that ε-NH_2 groups of lysine and hydroxylysine of collagen are directly involved in the interaction with the phosphate ion. The studies in which the ε-NH_2 groups were deaminated or modified with 1-fluoro-2,4-dinitrobenzene provided evidence that ε-NH_2 groups of lysine and hydroxylysine are in the immediate vicinity of the nucleation centres, but do not play any major role in the initiation of the nucleation process (GLIMCHER et al., 1965). The existence of "holes" in the collagen fibrils, which result from the quarter-stagger arrangement (cf. Fig. 2), makes it tempting to suppose that bone mineral is deposited in them (GLIMCHER et al., 1965). Recently, MARINO and BECKER (1967) provided evidence that a direct physical bond exists between the crystals of the initial mineralization phase and the collagen fibres.

Regulation of Mineralization

In the body, only the bone collagen has the property of inducing mineralization, though in vitro, collagens of other tissues exhibit a similar property (FLEISCH and NEUMAN, 1961). One of the differences between the nucleating and non-nucleating collagens might be the presence of some sort of inhibitor bound to the latter. This inhibitory substance was shown to be the inorganic pyrophosphate (FLEISCH and BISAZ, 1962), though this effect is a general property of polyphosphates (FLEISCH et al., 1966 a). It acts by blocking the nucleation centres, thus protecting the tissue against mineralization—while in mineralizing sites this inhibitor is destroyed by pyrophosphatase, providing for the liberation of the nucleating centre (FLEISCH and BISAZ, 1965).

The presence of pyrophosphate in tissues, mainly in the bone tissue, plasma, and urine, has been reported (FLEISCH and NEUMAN, 1961). The local pyrophosphate concentration may be the result of a dynamic equilibrium among the rates of its formation, destruction and excretion. Calcification may therefore be induced by a decrease in pyrophosphate production or an increase in pyrophosphatase concentration (FLEISCH and BISAZ, 1965).

Pyrophosphate, in addition to inhibiting mineralization, may also stabilize the amorphous calcium phosphate (BURLEY, 1965) and crystalline apatite (FLEISCH et al., 1966 a). Synthetic amorphous calcium phosphate transphosphorylates ATP into ADP and pyrophosphate, and becomes stabilized (BURLEY, 1965). The pyrophosphate ion was shown to have a high affinity for hydroxyapatite crystals, acting as some sort of buffer around these crystals, impeding their formation as well as their dissolution (FLEISCH et al., 1966).

Resorption of Bone Mineral

The close relation of calcium and collagen is the basis for similar resorption of both substances. LAITINEN (1967) provided evidence that mineral and collagen are removed almost simultaneously; the time courses of specific activity of urinary hydroxyproline and calcium after an injection of proline-^{14}C and ^{45}CaCl$_2$ were strikingly similar. The process of resorption is under the control of parathyroid hormone (PTH) and thyrocalcitonin (TCT).

A fall in the concentration of blood ionized calcium is the stimulus for PTH release (SHERWOOD et al., 1966). PTH stimulates bone resorption by inducing the cells of bone to revert to osteolytic cells (JOHNSTON et al., 1965; BAUD, 1966). Organic acids and proteolytic enzymes produced and secreted by bone cells are thought to be the agents of the solubilization of bone mineral (VAES, 1966; BAUD, 1966), and of the hydrolysis of collagen fibres (JOHNSTON et al., 1965; AVIOLI and PROCKOP, 1967). Ground substance is not hydrolyzed, but contrariwise, its synthesis is even increased (JOHNSTON et al., 1965). Parathyroidectomy does not produce any opposite metabolic effect to injection of PTH, but a general decrease in the metabolic activity of bone tissue, since, when PTH is removed, the lysis of bone followed by a secondary stimulation of new bone formation are both decreased (JOHNSTON et al., 1965).

PTH acts by control of gene activity. Actinomycin D, a specific inhibitor of DNA-dependent synthesis of complementary RNA (a transcription inhibitor), injected prior to parathyroid extract blocks its action (RASMUSSEN et al., 1964; RAISZ and NIEMANN, 1966). Vitamin D is necessary for physiologic concentrations of PTH to mobilize bone mineral (ARNAUD et al., 1966).

An elevation in the concentration of blood ionized calcium is the stimulus for thyrocalcitonin release (MACINTYRE et al., 1964). Present evidence suggests that TCT is produced by the parafollicular cells (thyroid C cells) of the thyroid gland (O'RIORDAN, 1967). The major site of action of TCT is bone, where it inhibits bone resorption (SOLIMAN et al., 1966; KLEIN and TALMAGE, 1968). WASE et al. (1967) provided evidence suggesting that TCT, continuously administered over a long period of time, enhances cortical bone development. The effectiveness of TCT in parathyroidectomized rats showed that it need not act by blocking secretion of PTH (MUNSON, 1966). Marked effects of thyrocalcitonin in the presence of increased levels of parathyroid hormone indicate that the former blocks the effects of the later upon bone resorption (ANAST et al., 1967; KLEIN and TALMAGE, 1968).

Thyrocalcitonin neither acts by control of gene activity (actinomycin D injected prior to calcitonin does not block its action) nor is its activity dependent on vitamin D (SOLIMAN et al., 1966).

Chapter 2

General Outlines
of a Clinical Approach to Bone Tissue Metabolism

The content of mineral relative to organic matrix in bone is remarkably constant under physiological and most pathological conditions, since bone tissue is being formed and resorbed in toto (BAUER et al., 1961). Theoretically, there should be no difference in quantifying the bone tissue metabolism, irrespective of whether the bone mineral or the organic matrix is studied. In practice, at least in man, only the bone calcium metabolism is readily available for quantitative measurements, owing to the lack of any significant calcium stores besides the skeleton that could influence the overall metabolism of this element (HEANEY, 1964). On the other hand, it is practically impossible to measure the bone metabolism of inorganic phosphate, the counter ion of calcium, since the large amounts of organic tissue phosphates strongly interfere (BAUER et al., 1961).

Also the metabolism of bone matrix cannot be strictly quantified, owing to interference of collagen from other stores of connective tissue. Hence, the urinary excretion of hydroxyproline is assumed to be an index only, and not the measure, of bone collagen metabolism (PROCKOP and KIVIRIKKO, 1967). The same goes for the urinary excretion of pyrophosphate, the anion regulating the process of mineralization (FLEISCH et al., 1966).

Some of the most important features of calcium metabolism (plasma state, renal handling, net absorption and faecal output), the major features of phosphate metabolism (plasma state and renal handling), and the urinary excretion of hydroxyproline and pyrophosphate—may be investigated by conventional techniques. The remaining data of prime importance, that is, the rates of new bone formation and bone resorption, the true absorption of calcium in the gastrointestinal tract, and the excretion of endogenous calcium in faeces—cannot be obtained by these techniques and require the application of methods making use of tracers. Tracer methodology depends on the assumption that the atoms of the injected isotope of calcium, or any other tracer, behave exactly like the atoms of natural element, the tracee (BROWNELL et al., 1968), and that the system under study cannot discriminate between them (SOLOMON, 1960).

1. Calcium Metabolism

The major pathways of calcium metabolism may be outlined as in Fig. 8.

A fraction of the ingested calcium is absorbed in the small intestine, and the remainder passes through the gastrointestinal tract and is excreted in the faeces without having been absorbed. Similarly, of the calcium secreted with the digestive juices, a fraction is reabsorbed, and the remainder appears in the faeces. Calcium

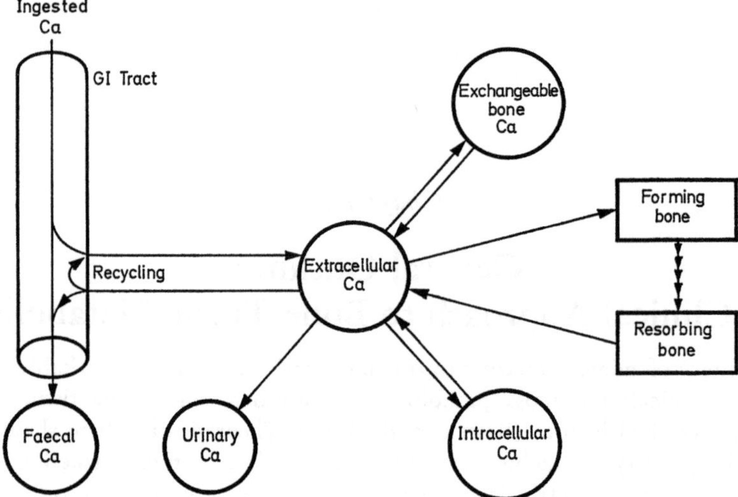

Fig. 8. General scheme of calcium metabolism. The gastrointestinal (GI) tract, exchangeable calcium in extracellular fluid, cells and bone, and nonexchangeable calcium in bone are represented

circulating in body fluids is maintained at a constant level in equilibrium with its levels in the intracellular fluid and in the exchangeable bone mineral. Calcium is accreted in bone tissue in the process of new bone formation or remodelling, and resorbed from bone tissue in the process of bone destruction. The loss of endogenous calcium in the urine and faeces is compensated for by an equivalent intake of this element.

Calcium Absorption

The fate of calcium in the gastrointestinal tract is indicated in Fig. 9.

Daily ingested calcium V_i and that entering the gut with digestive juices V_d, both being only partially absorbed from the intestinal lumen, add to the unabsorbed element that appears in faeces V_F. The difference between the rates of intake and faecal output, the net absorption rate $V_{a\,(net)}$, is given by the formula:

$$V_{a\,(net)} = V_i - V_F \, . \tag{1}$$

It may be obtained by simple determination of calcium in the food and faeces sampled on a time basis, that is, over an appropriate balance periode timed with time-markers (REIFENSTEIN et al., 1945).

By subtracting the excretion rate of endogenous faecal calcium V_f from the excretion rate of total faecal calcium, the excretion rate of exogenous faecal calcium $\beta\,V_i$ is obtained:

$$\beta\,V_i = F_F - V_f \, . \tag{2}$$

The endogenous faecal calcium denotes calcium secreted into the gut with digestive juices and then excreted in the faeces, excluding that secreted into the gut and then reabsorbed. The excretion rate of endogenous faecal calcium is calculated from the amount of tracer excreted in faeces following its intravenous administration, since, being administered intravenously, all tracer in faeces is endogenous. Assuming the

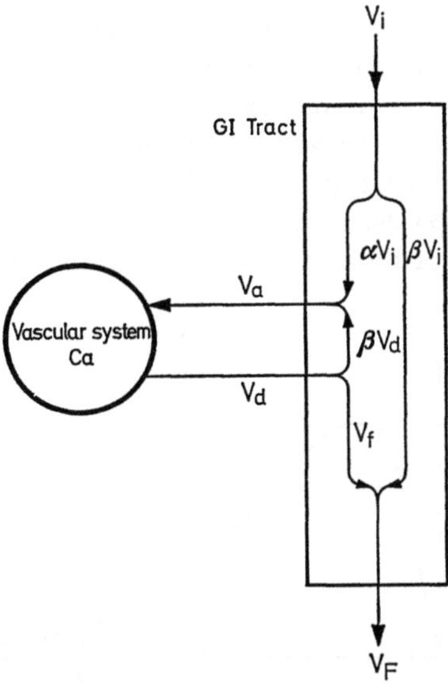

Fig. 9. General relations between absorption of ingested and digestive juice calcium and excretion of endogenous and exogenous faecal calcium

specific activity of calcium secreted into the gut and excreted in urine at the same time interval to be identical, the excretion rate of endogenous faecal calcium may be obtained by the formula of AUBERT and MILHAUD (1960):

$$V_f = V_u \frac{f_{faeces}}{f_{urine}} \tag{3}$$

where V_u = excretion rate of urinary calcium, f_{faeces} = fraction of tracer excreted in faeces, and f_{urine} = fraction excreted in urine, both accurately timed with a correction for faecal lag (cf. Fig. 23).

The difference between the ingested calcium and the exogenous faecal calcium is the true absorption rate V_a (BRONNER et al., 1962):

$$V_a = V_i - \beta V_i. \tag{4}$$

Calcium secreted into the gut and then reabsorbed cannot be obtained in vivo, since its fractional reabsorption rate βV_d is not observable even with the aid of isotopes (MARSHALL, 1964).

The rate of entry of the radioisotope from the intestinal tract into the vascular system is usually given as the integrated steady state rate of absorption from the entire gut. Recently, HART and SPENCER (1967) studied the initial entry rate of the tracer, i. e. entry of the tracer from one compartment into another compartment of the system, without consideration of recirculation or feedback; this reflects the gradual passage of the remaining unabsorbed dose of tracer through different portions of the intestinal tract, exhibiting different transport activity (HART and SPENCER, 1967). The appearance of the tracer in the vascular space can be expressed by the Volterra integral equation:

$$G(t) = \int_0^t B(\tau) F(t-\tau) \, d\tau \tag{5}$$

in which G(t) is the plasma activity curve following an oral tracer dose at time $t_0 = 0$; B(τ) is the rate of initial entry at time τ following an oral tracer dose, at which the tracer first appears in the vascular system; F(t) is the plasma activity curve following intravenous tracer administration (HART and SPENCER, 1967). Since G(t) and F(t) are determined experimentally, the integral equation can be solved by standard means, and B(τ) determined either analytically (BERKOWITZ et al., 1963; HART and SPENCER, 1967) or by a computer (HART and SPENCER, 1967).

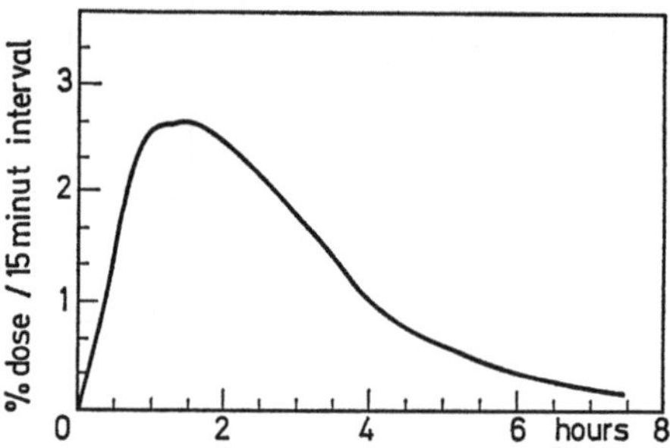

Fig. 10. Rate of initial entry of radiocalcium from the intestine into the vascular space. (From HART and SPENCER, 1967)

Fig. 10 illustrates a typical result for the initial entry functions from the intestine into the vascular system for 15 minutes intervals employed in the calculations (HART and SPENCER, 1967). The integrated area under the curve gives the cumulative absorption for tracer, identical with that obtained in above test on true absorption.

Detailed studies on the transport of calcium across the intestinal wall have led to the conclusion that calcium absorption is not due solely to passive diffusion, but that there is an active transport system with a maximal absorptive capacity maintained by vitamin D. This vitamin acts in the mucosal epithelial cell, inducing the biosynthesis of a carrier which facilitates the movement of calcium across the intestinal mucosa. The vitamin D-induced calcium-binding factor was isolated from chicks (WASSERMAN and TAYLOR, 1963; TAYLOR and WASSERMAN, 1965) and rats (KALLFELTZ et al., 1967). This is a protein whose synthesis may be inhibited by actinomycin D (TAYLOR and WASSERMAN, 1965). In the intact animal, the calcium-binding protein may possibly act as an intracellular carrier for calcium, increasing the movement of this element back and forth across the intestinal mucosal cell (KALLFELTZ et al., 1967).

Calcium in Body Fluids

Bone tissue shares an internal environment with the other tissues of the body (McLEAN and BUDY, 1964). This environment, that is, the extracellular fluid, includes the blood plasma and the interstitial fluid.

Total plasma calcium exists in two major fractions of roughly equal size: non-diffusible or protein-bound, and diffusible or non-protein-bound (ultrafiltrable) calcium. The diffusible fraction is further distributed between ionized and complexed, mainly citrate linked, calcium (WALSER, 1961). The state of calcium in normal plasma is presented in Fig. 11.

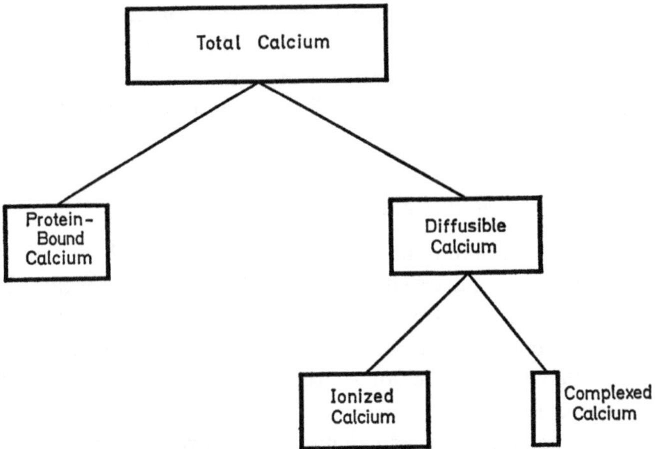

Fig. 11. The state of calcium in normal plasma

The affinity of the plasma proteins for calcium may be expressed by a simple dissociation constant of calcium proteinate K_{CaProt} given by the equation:

$$K_{CaProt} = \frac{[Ca^{2+}] \cdot [Proteinate^{2-}]}{[Ca\ Proteinate]} \qquad (6)$$

where $[Ca^{2+}]$ is the concentration of ionized calcium, and $[Proteinate^{2-}]$ is the concentration of protein, both expressed as moles per liter (McLEAN and HASTINGS, 1935). Since the ultrafiltration data are used in calculating the dissociation constant of calcium proteinate and all the plasma proteins are considered together, the following formula may be used:

$$K_{CaProt} = \frac{[Ca]_{UF}\ ([Protein] - [Ca\ Proteinate])}{[Ca\ Proteinate]} \qquad (7)$$

and $$[Ca\ Proteinate] = [Ca]_P - [Ca]_{UF}$$

where $[Ca]_P$ and $[Ca]_{UF}$ represent plasma and ultrafiltrate concentrations of calcium, respectively, in moles per liter, and [Protein] represents protein concentration, also in moles per liter (the product of $1.22 \cdot 10^{-3}$ and protein concentration in g per 100 ml) (WALSER, 1962).

For calculating the concentration of diffusible calcium in plasma from ultrafiltration data, a formula should be used which makes allowance for plasma water and the Donnan factor for divalent cations:

$$[Ca]_D = (0.990 - 0.008\ [Protein]) \cdot [Ca]_{UF}\ 1.05 \qquad (8)$$

where $[Ca]_D$ is the concentration of diffusible calcium in plasma, $[Ca]_{UF}$ is the concentration of calcium in ultrafiltrate, [Protein] is the concentration of plasma proteins expressed in grams per cent, and 1.05 is the Donnan factor for calcium. In practice, in calculating the concentration of diffusible calcium in plasma, both the correction for plasma water and the Donnan factor may be omitted, since in the case of divalent cations the two corrections are opposite in direction and of approximately equal magnitude. Thus, the concentration of calcium in ultrafiltrate is equal to the concentration of diffusible calcium in native plasma.

The diffusible calcium, which approximates that in protein-poor interstitial fluid, is in dynamic equilibrium throughout the body with continuous exchange among the compartments of the exchangeable calcium system. The latter, besides plasma and interstitial fluid calcium, comprises also cell calcium and exchangeable bone calcium (RICH, 1961; HEANEY, 1964).

Renal Handling of Calcium

The renal handling of calcium may be sketched as in Fig. 12.

Only the diffusible plasma calcium is filtered at the glomerulus. From the diffusible plasma calcium that passes the glomerular filter, about 95—99 per cent is reabsorbed. Reabsorption of the filtered calcium takes place along the entire nephron (LASSITER et al., 1963). The calcium excreted in the urine is the non-reabsorbed fraction of the filtered load.

In tests of the renal handling of calcium, the concentration of diffusible plasma calcium given by formula (8) should be corrected for the fractional plasma water content and the Donnan factor, since the diffusible calcium in the protein-free phase of native plasma is distributed across the semipermeable glomerulus membrane in accordance with this factor. But both corrections may be omitted in calculations based on plasma ultrafiltrate. Thus, either the product of diffusible plasma calcium concentration, the fractional plasma water content, and the Donnan factor of $1:1.05 = 0.95$, or the concentration of calcium in plasma ultrafiltrate, may be used in calculations.

The simplest expression for renal handling of calcium is the renal clearance of calcium C_{Ca} given by the formula:

$$C_{Ca} = \frac{Ca_U \, V}{Ca_{UF}} \tag{9}$$

where Ca_{UF} and Ca_U represent the concentrations of calcium in plasma ultrafiltrate and urine, respectively, in amount of calcium per 1 ml, and V is the diuresis in ml per minute. The product $Ca_U V$ is the urinary calcium excretion per minute. The renal clearance of calcium, expressed as the volume of filtrate cleared per minute, does not give any closer insight into the discrete processes of renal handling of calcium: the filtered load and the tubular reabsorption of calcium.

The filtered load of calcium FL_{Ca} is simply the product of calcium concentration in 1 ml of plasma ultrafiltrate and the volume of filtrate produced per minute in the glomeruli (termed true glomerular filtration rate) GFR:

$$FL_{Ca} = Ca_{UF} \, GFR \, . \tag{10}$$

It is expressed as the quantity of calcium filtered per minute.

The tubular reabsorption of calcium T_{Ca} is the difference between the filtered calcium and that excreted in the urine:

$$T_{Ca} = FL_{Ca} - Ca_U \, V \tag{11}$$

and represents the amount of calcium reabsorbed per minute. But it may be also expressed as the quantity of calcium reabsorbed per 100 ml glomerular filtrate, $100 \, T_{Ca}/GFR$, and as a percentage of the filtered load of calcium, $\% \, T_{Ca} = 100 \, T_{Ca}/FL_{Ca}$. The latter expression is of great practical significance.

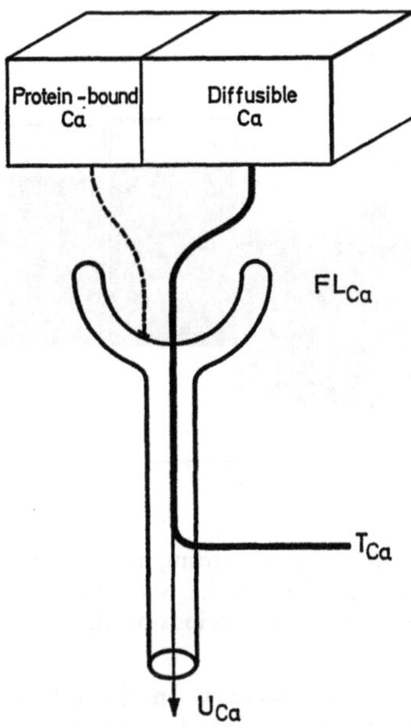

Fig. 12. Renal handling of calcium. FL$_{Ca}$ = filtered calcium; T$_{Ca}$ = tubular reabsorption of calcium; U$_{Ca}$ = urinary calcium

Bone Calcium Accretion and Resorption

Bone is constantly being formed and resorbed (BAUER et al., 1961). When the skeleton does not change its shape or size, the rates of new bone formation and resorption balance each other—owing to the continual adaptation of the skeleton to its environment, referred to as the remodelling of bones. The overall balance between bone mineral formation and resorption is reflected in the difference between the intake and excretion of calcium, since any distinct change in calcium balance indicates a change in bone, owing to the fact that over 99 per cent of body calcium is deposited in bone.

Metabolic balance studies require complete and accurately timed estimates of the intake of calcium in the diet and its excretion in urine and faeces. The balance data obtained, expressed according to the convention of REIFENSTEIN et al. (1945), are presented in Fig. 13.

The daily intake of calcium is plotted downwards from the base-line. For the relevant periods, the faecal calcium is plotted above the intake line, and the urinary calcium above the faecal line. The difference between the base-line and the upper line of excretion is the balance: positive when the upper line of excretion remains below the base-line; zero when it lies on the base-line; and negative when it exceeds the base-line.

It is relatively simple to measure the dietary and urinary calcium and relate the collection of urine to the diet consumed. Two methods are employed for quantitative faecal collections: the time-marker method and the inert-marker method. In the former, a time marker is given orally at the start of a metabolic balance study and repeated at appropriate balance periods for the next few weeks (LUTWAK and BURTON, 1964). Faeces excreted between the time of appearance in the faeces of the first and second markers is related to the diet consumed and the urine voided in the

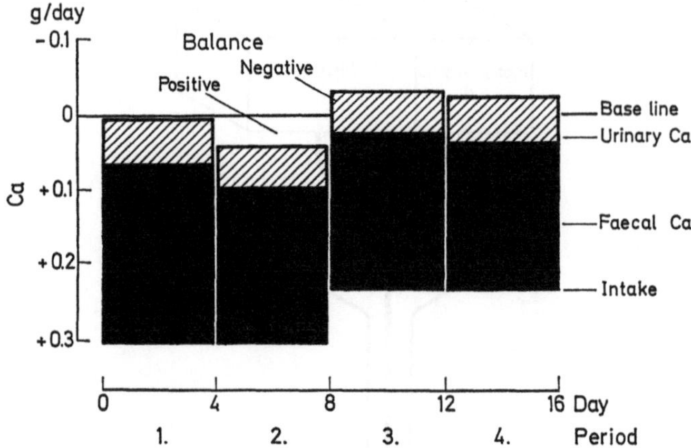

Fig. 13. Calcium balance data expressed according to the convention of Reifenstein et al. (1945). Base-line study on 305 mg calcium intake is shown in two periods on the left, and on 235 mg calcium intake is shown in two periods on the right. Case Z.A., osteoporosis

interval between the giving of the markers. In the latter, the doses of inert-marker are taken with the main meals. The excretion of inert marker indicates the completeness of faecal collections and permits corrections for variations in faecal passage (Stanley and Cheng, 1957). Used for these purposes are: chromic oxide (Whitby and Lang, 1960; Davignon et al., 1968), ^{51}Cr-labelled haemoglobin, and ^{47}Sc (Pearson, 1966).

If bone resorption is equal to bone formation, the balance of calcium is very near to zero. If resorption predominates over formation of bone and the skeleton loses calcium, the calcium balance is negative. If bone formation predominates over bone resorption and the skeleton accumulates calcium, the calcium balance is positive. Hence, the bone accretion of calcium minus the relative value of calcium balance gives the resorption of bone calcium (Heaney, 1964).

The study of the rate of calcium accretion cannot be carried out by conventional techniques and requires the use of tracer kinetics.

Application of Tracer Kinetics to Calcium Metabolism

Body calcium represents two distinct and essentially independent moieties: an exchangeable and a nonexchangeable calcium pool. The latter is present mainly in the bone. In tracer kinetics, the exchangeable calcium pool, called a system, is regarded as being composed of a finite number of discrete states, called compartments, and as having uniform specific activity within each state (Brownell et al., 1968). This system is open to a source (food calcium, resorbing bone calcium) and to a sink of calcium (urinary calcium, endogenous faecal calcium, accreted calcium). The open calcium system is in a steady-state when the amount of this element in each compartment and the flow rates between the compartments remain constant with time, and the loss of calcium by the system is exactly compensated by calcium entering it.

To study the calcium system, a first-order perturbation is introduced by the use of calcium tracer, that is, too little to affect the system significantly, yet enough to be measurable. Since, even within a nonlinear system, the response of a tracer is always linear, linear kinetics may be applied to the interpretation of data from studies on calcium metabolism with the aid of tracers (BERMAN, 1968). To interpret data from such studies, a formal description of the system is needed: a physical model which is a simplified description of the system represented by its mathematical formalism and compatible with the experimental observations. The physical model consists of a set of compartments with interconnections, and the mathematical formalism for the description of this model is a set of linear differential equations with constant coefficients (BROWNELL et al., 1968).

Early in the studies on calcium kinetics, the noncompartmental method had been used, but nowadays the multicompartmental analysis of calcium kinetics is preferred, employing two, three and four exchanging compartments in the system. It is not possible to choose among the different models—each one being an operational entity useful to describe the system. Fortunately, certain parameters of special interest are the external components of the system, and hence, they are not too much dependent on the particular model. These parameters are the rates of renal excretion, endogenous faecal excretion, and bone accretion of calcium.

The simplest method, fairly consistent with the experimental data, was the noncompartmental method of BAUER et al. (1955). The conceptual basis upon which the use of this method rested was presented by CARLSSON (1951): bone represents an exchangeable calcium fraction in which tracer concentration parallels that of the body fluids and the nonexchangeable calcium, into which the tracer is irreversibly deposited in the process of bone accretion. Hence, at any time following its introduction into the plasma, the specific activity of a tracer can be separated conceptually into two fractions, the first changing in proportion to the plasma calcium specific activity X_P and the second in proportion to the time integral of X_P (MARSHALL, 1964). The body retention of tracer R may be given by the equation developed by BAUER, CARLSSON and LINDQUIST (1955):

$$R = EX_P + (V_0^+ + V_u + V_f) \int_0^t X_P(t)\, dt \qquad (12)$$

where E is the amount of calcium in the exchangeable system, and V_0^+, V_u, and V_f are the rates of bone accretion, urinary excretion, and faecal endogenous excretion of calcium, respectively. The use of the BCL method has to be restricted to a certain time interval: longer than the time needed for uniform distribution of tracer throughout the exchangeable pool, that is, longer than the mixing phase of tracer, usually equal to 2 days, yet short enough to preclude the influence of resorption, that is, shorter than the time needed for recycling of the accreted tracer. Moreover, this method does not give any insight into the compartments of the system, but is fairly valid for the turnover rate of the system, i. e. the estimate of the fraction of calcium that leaves the system per unit time. The external components of the turnover rate could be determined by measurement of tracer and tracee in the excreta (urine and faeces). The difference between the total turnover rate and the excretion rate of calcium has been attributed to internal loss of calcium in the process of new bone formation (BAUER et al., 1955; HEANEY and WHEDON, 1958; AUBERT and MILHAUD, 1960). This approach leads to an overestimation of the pool size as well as of the bone accretion rate (HEANEY, 1964; MARSHALL, 1964). Nevertheless, it has been the conceptual basis for measurement of calcium accretion.

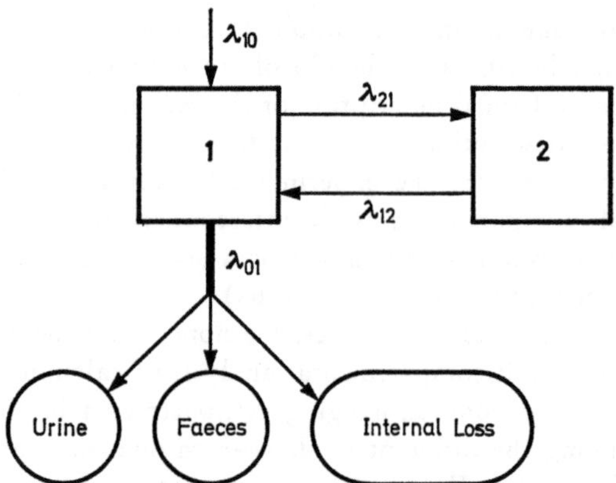

Fig. 14. Two-compartmental open system model of calcium turnover compatible with a two-exponential plasma disappearance curve of calcium tracer. Compartment 1 represents the pool of calcium in isotopic equilibrium within a few hours. Compartment 2 represents the pool of calcium in isotopic equilibrium within two days. λ_{ij} are the fractional rate constants of calcium transfer into compartment i from compartment j; λ_{10} is the fractional rate constant of calcium entry into the system; λ_{01} is the fractional rate constant of unidirectional calcium loss, and includes the urinary excretion, faecal endogenous calcium excretion, and internal loss to nonexchanging bone

A better approach is the two-compartment system method advocated by HEANEY (1964). The structure of this system, the two-compartment model presented in Fig. 14, reflects the transient phenomena occurring after the injection of tracer into the blood: the rapid mixing of tracer within a large nonskeletal exchanging compartment, Compartment 1, and the slower mixing of tracer within the skeletal compartment, Compartment 2. The activity lost to the outside by urinary excretion and faecal excretion subtracted from the activity lost from Compartment 1 reflects the internal loss of activity, that is, the activity taken up by bone. Hence, the turnover-difference concept is still valid. The analytical solution of this model has been presented by HEANEY (1964), and the solution by computer by COHN et al. (1965). To use this model, the plasma disappearance curve of calcium tracer, obtained at times of less than 4 hours, should be excluded.

The plasma disappearance curve of calcium tracer obtained at times of more than 20 minutes—that is, longer than the time needed for mixing the tracer in the physiologically active part of the extracellular fluid (SZYMENDERA et al., 1966)—fits a sum of three exponentials. Thus, at least three compartments are required for the exchangeable calcium system. The three-compartment mammillary system model and its solution by the computer has been presented by AVIOLI and HENNEMAN (1964). This model, used in this study, is presented in Chapter 3, and its analytical solution is given in Appendix.

Recently NEER et al. (1967) introduced the four-compartment system model, presented in Fig. 15, for studying the kinetics of calcium. The internal loss of calcium into forming bone takes place from the fourth compartment, and the loss of calcium into the urine and faeces from the first. This model is useful for some types of study: for studying the coordinated regulatory responses in intact man. This model, called

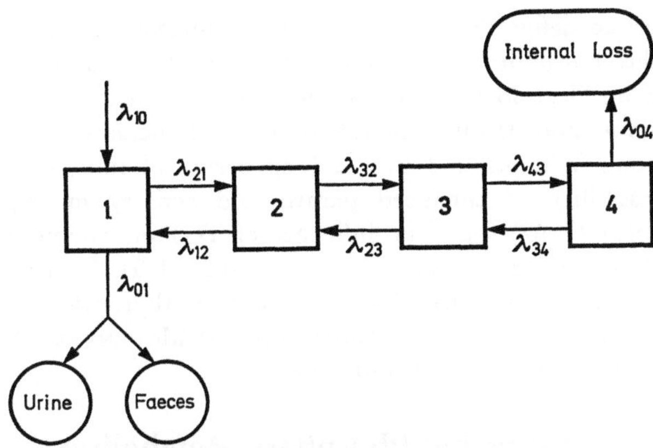

Fig. 15. Open series four-compartment system model of calcium turnover compatible with a four-exponential plasma disappearance curve of calcium tracer. Compartments 1—4 are operational entities, useful to describe and analyze the system. The fractional rate constants λ_{ij} represent transfer of calcium between compartments, loss of calcium to urine and faeces and internal loss into nonexchanging bone

therefore the regulatory model, includes the plasma disappearance curve of calcium tracer obtained at times of less than 20 minutes; in practice, from the beginning to 7 days after the injection of tracer.

Skeletal Hormones and Calcium Metabolism

Parathyroid hormone (PTH) and thyrocalcitonin (TCT) are the two parts of a dual hormonal mechanism in the homeostatic regulation of ionized calcium concentration in the blood plasma. The concentration of ionized calcium in the plasma is itself the stimulus to which the parathyroid glands and the parafollicular cells of the thyroid gland respond; thus, the condition being regulated activates the regulatory mechanism, which is a negative feedback in terms of control system theory (McLean and Budy, 1964).

A fall in the concentration of blood ionized calcium is the stimulus for PTH release. The released parathyroid hormone starts to control calcium homeostasis by coordinated stimulatory effects of approximately equal magnitude on gut, bone, and kidney (Phang et al., 1967). Thus, PTH increases the absorption of calcium in the small intestine (Cramer, 1963; Care and Keynes, 1964), the resorption of bone (cf. Chapter 1, part 3), and the tubular reabsorption of calcium (Kleeman et al., 1958; Bernstein et al., 1963; Transbøl et al., 1968). The result is that the concentration of ionized calcium in blood plasma rises and shuts off the secretion of hormone.

The role of thyrocalcitonin is to prevent an overshooting of the upper borderline in concentration of plasma ionized calcium following PTH release. Ionized calcium hypercalcaemia is the stimulus for TCT release. The released thyrocalcitonin controls calcium homeostasis by inhibiting the catabolism of bone, which is the main mechanism involved in the lowering of the plasma calcium concentration (Milhaud and Moukhtar, 1966 b; Anast et al., 1967). TCT inhibits the action of PTH on bone resorption, as well as inhibiting bone resorption in the absence of PTH (Kohler and Pechet, 1966; Carroll and Pechet, 1967; Klein et al., 1967). The studies undertaken in an effort to define the effect of TCT on intestinal calcium transport have not ruled out this possibility: CARE and KEYNES (1964) found decreased calcium absorption from an ileal loop in one sheep after intravenous injection of thyrocalcitonin; MILHAUD and MOUKHTAR (1966 b) found increased calcium absorption after thyrocalcitonin administered over a long period of time, but they could not rule out the possibility of enhanced parathyroid activity in response to hypocalcaemia; KRAWITT (1967) found no influence of TCT on calcium transport in the rat duodenum. It might be concluded that the effect of TCT on intestinal calcium transport is either small or none. Also the effect of thyrocalcitonin on the renal handling of calcium is still unknown (MILHAUD and MOUKHTAR, 1966 a; MILHAUD and MOUKHTAR, 1966 b; RASMUSSEN et al., 1967).

2. Inorganic Phosphate Metabolism

The major pathways of inorganic phosphate metabolism resemble those of calcium metabolism, though quantitatively they differ in several points, as shown in Fig. 16.

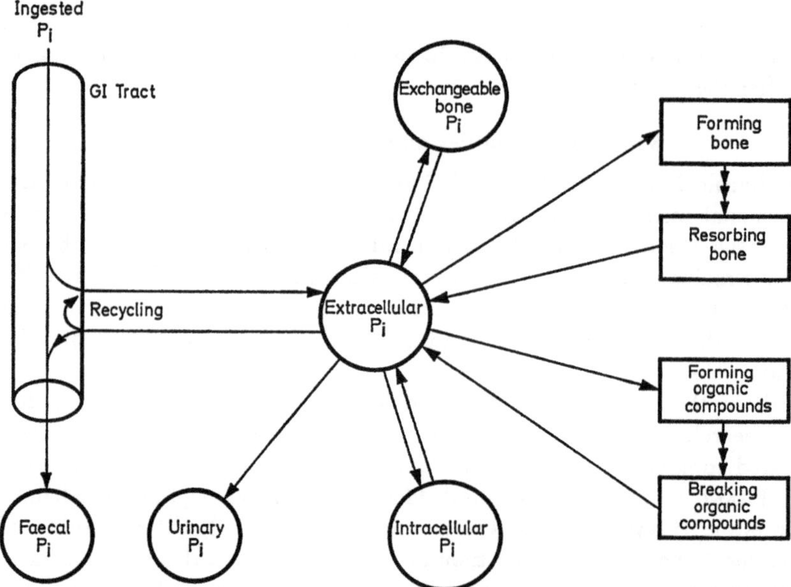

Fig. 16. General scheme of inorganic phosphate metabolism. The gastrointestinal (GI) tract, exchangeable phosphate in extracellular fluid, cells and bone, and nonexchangeable phosphate in bone and organic compounds of long half-life are represented

The greater part of the ingested phosphate is absorbed in the small intestine, and the remaining small fraction is excreted in the faeces. Similarly, of the quantity of phosphate secreted with the digestive juices, a fraction is reabsorbed, and the remainder appears in the faeces. Inorganic phosphate circulating in body fluids is in equilibrium with that in intracellular fluid and in the exchangeable bone mineral. The major fraction of soft tissue phosphate is present in an organic form, while that of bone phosphate is in the inorganic form. Phosphate is accreted into bone tissue in the process of new bone formation or remodelling, and resorbed from it in the process of bone destruction. In addition, phosphate is transformed into a number of organic components having a life span not shorter than that of bone mineral. The loss of endogenous phosphate in urine, and about one tenth of this in faeces, is compensated for by an equivalent intake of this ion.

Owing to the vast complexity of phosphate metabolism, only the plasma state and renal handling of inorganic phosphate are routinely studied, whereas the kinetics of inorganic phosphate metabolism is investigated on exceptional occasions only.

Phosphate in Body Fluids

The internal environment of the body tissues includes the extracellular fluid, that is, the blood plasma and the interstitial fluid.

Total plasma inorganic phosphate exists in two fractions: non-diffusible or protein-bound, and diffusible or nonprotein-bound (ultrafiltrable) phosphate. The diffusible fraction distributes further between ionized and complexed (with calcium and magnesium) phosphate (WALSER, 1961). The state of inorganic phosphate in normal plasma is presented in Fig. 17.

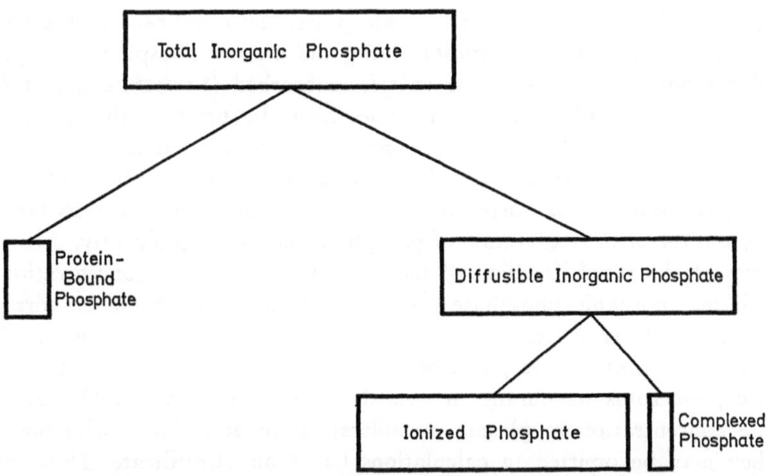

Fig. 17. The state of inorganic phosphate in normal plasma

For calculating the concentration of diffusible inorganic phosphate from ultrafiltration data, a formula should be used which makes allowance for plasma water and the Donnan factor for phosphate ions in plasma:

$$[P_i]_D = (0.990 - 0.008\,[\text{Protein}]) \cdot [P_i]_{UF} \cdot 0.915 \tag{13}$$

where $[P_i]_D$ is the concentration of diffusible phosphate in plasma, $[P_i]_{UF}$ is the concentration of phosphate in ultrafiltrate, [Protein] is the concentration of plasma proteins expressed in grams per cent, and 0.915 is the Donnan factor for phosphate (WALSER, 1960; WALSER, 1961).

The plasma diffusible inorganic phosphate is in the form of ions and complexes: $H_2PO_4^-$ (10 per cent), $NaHPO_4^-$ (29 per cent), HPO_4^{2-} (43 per cent), $CaHPO_4$ (3 per cent), and $MgHPO_4$ (3 per cent) (WALSER, 1961).

The rest of the plasma inorganic phosphate, about 12 per cent, is protein-bound. For calculating the protein-bound phosphate, the concentrations of total inorganic phosphate and diffusible inorganic phosphate in native plasma should be used. Thus, the percentage of protein-bound inorganic plasma phosphate may be calculated according to the formula:

$$\% \, P_{\text{protein-bound}} = 100 \, (1 - [P_i]_D/[P_i]_P) \tag{14}$$

where $[P_i]_P$ is the concentration of total inorganic phosphate in native plasma.

The plasma phosphate concentration varies according to time of day and phosphate intake. Tests that involve the plasma and urinary phosphate must be done under strictly standardized conditions. ANNINO and RELMAN (1958) have shown that an ordinary breakfast lowers plasma phosphate concentration by about 30 per cent within 45 minutes after eating; this concentration returns to the fasting value within 2 hours. The restriction of phosphorus in the diet also lowers the level of phosphate in plasma, but for longer periods of time.

Renal Handling of Phosphate

The renal handling of phosphate may be sketched as in Fig. 18.

Only the diffusible inorganic phosphate passes the membrane of the glomerular tuft (WALSER, 1960). Of the diffusible inorganic plasma phosphate that passes the glomerular filter, about 78—94 per cent is reabsorbed (SZYMENDERA and MADAJEWICZ, in press). The phosphate that passes into the urine is the non-reabsorbed fraction of the filtered load; on an ordinary diet the normal adult excretes in the urine about 600 mg phosphate per day. When intestinal absorption of phosphates is reduced, the tubular reabsorption of filtered phosphate may rise so far as to be complete, and the urinary excretion of phosphate may fall significantly.

In tests of the renal handling of inorganic phosphate, the concentration of diffusible plasma inorganic phosphate given by formula (13) should be corrected for the fractional plasma water content and the Donnan factor, since the diffusible phosphate in the protein-free phase of native plasma is distributed across the semipermeable glomerulus membrane in accordance with this factor. However, as the phosphate concentration in plasma ultrafiltrate is in accordance with both corrections, they may be omitted in calculations based on ultrafiltrate. Thus, either the product of diffusible inorganic phosphate concentration, the fractional plasma water content, and the Donnan factor of $1:0.915 = 1.09$, or the concentration of inorganic phosphate in plasma ultrafiltrate may be used in calculations.

The simplest expression for renal handling of inorganic phosphate is the renal clearance of phosphate C_P given by the formula:

$$C_P = \frac{P_U \, V}{P_{UF}} \tag{15}$$

where P_{UF} and P_U represent the concentration of inorganic phosphate per ml plasma ultrafiltrate and urine, respectively, and V is the diuresis in ml per minute. The product $P_U \, V$ is the urinary phosphate excretion per minute. The renal clearance of inorganic phosphate, expressed as the volume of filtrate cleared per minute, does not give any closer insight into the two processes involved: the filtered load and the tubular reabsorption of inorganic phosphate.

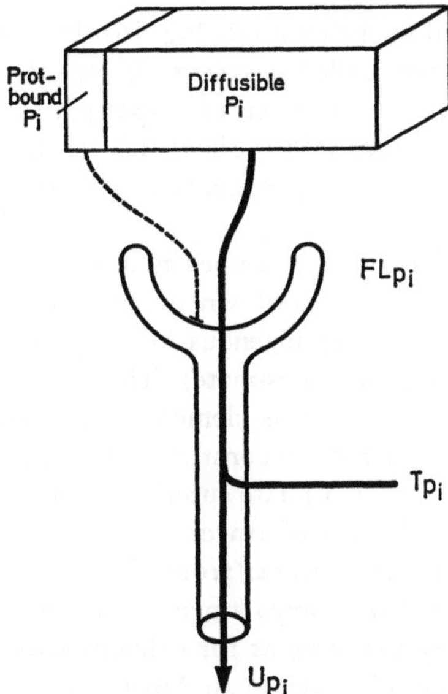

Fig. 18. Renal handling of phosphate. FL$_{Pi}$ = filtered inorganic phosphate; T$_{Pi}$ = tubular reabsorption of inorganic phosphate; U$_{Pi}$ = inorganic urinary phosphate

The filtered load of inorganic phosphate FL$_P$ is simply the product of inorganic phosphate concentration in 1 ml of plasma ultrafiltrate and the volume of filtrate produced per minute in the glomeruli (termed true glomerular filtration rate)[1] GFR:

$$FL_P = P_{UF} \, GFR . \tag{16}$$

It is expressed as the amount of inorganic phosphate filtered per minute.

The tubular reabsorption of phosphate T$_P$ is the difference between the filtered phosphate and that excreted in urine:

$$T_P = FL_P - P_U V \tag{17}$$

and represents the quantity of phosphate reabsorbed per minute. It may be also expressed as the quantity of phosphate reabsorbed per 100 ml glomerular filtrate, 100 T$_P$/GFR, and as a percentage of the filtered load of inorganic phosphate, $\% \, T_P = 100 \, T_P / FL_P$.

The renal handling of phosphate is the most important control for plasma concentration of inorganic phosphate (IRVING, 1964).

Application of Tracer Kinetics to Phosphate Metabolism

Body phosphate represents three distinct and essentially independent moieties: an exchangeable inorganic phosphate pool in extracellular fluid, cells and bone; an exchangeable phosphate pool in organic compounds of long life span; and a non-

---

[1] To obtain the true glomerular filtration from the creatinine clearance, defined as Cr$_U$V/Cr$_P$, in which Cr$_U$ and Cr$_P$ are urinary and plasma concentrations of creatinine, respectively, and V is urine volume per minute, the C$_{Cr}$ must be multiplied by the fractional plasma water content.

exchangeable phosphate pool in skeleton (cf. Fig. 16). In tracer kinetics, the exchange-able inorganic phosphate pool, called a system, is regarded as being composed of a finite number of compartments. LAX et al. (1956) assumed a system containing 15 compartments, but GESCHWIND (1961) showed in normal and hypophysectomized rats that a system containing 3 compartments is a better approximation of experi-mental data.

The exchangeable phosphate system is open to a source (food phosphate, resorbing bone phosphate, phosphate from breakdown of organic compounds), and to a sink of phosphate (urinary phosphate, endogenous faecal phosphate, bone-forming phos-phate, organic compound-forming phosphate). The open system of phosphate is in a steady state, when the amount of this element in each compartment and the flow rates between the compartments remain constant with time, and the loss of phosphate by the system is compensated by phosphate entering it (cf. Fig. 16).

To study this system by the aid of tracers, the same approach as for calcium is applied. Since the disappearance of tracer from plasma follows a curve composed of three exponentials, at least a three-compartment system model is required. The model used in this study, essentially the same as for calcium kinetics, is presented in Chap-ter 3, and its analytical solution is given in an Appendix.

Skeletal Hormones and Phosphate Metabolism

The homeostasis of plasma inorganic phosphate is much harder to explain than that of plasma calcium, since, contrary to the situation with respect to calcium, the inorganic phosphate concentration in plasma, the condition being regulated, has not been shown to be the stimulus to which any of the endocrine glands responds (McLEAN and BUDY, 1964).

Although parathyroid hormone and thyrocalcitonin have antagonistic effects upon bone tissue and plasma calcium (cf. Chapter 1, part 3), they both lower plasma phosphate (HIRSCH et al., 1964; MILHAUD and MOUKHTAR, 1966 a; ANAST et al., 1967; RASMUSSEN et al., 1967) and induce phosphaturia (MILHAUD and MOUKHTAR, 1966 a; ANAST et al., 1967; RASMUSSEN et al., 1967).

Parathyroid hormone lowers plasma phosphate affecting precisely the kidneys, markedly decreasing the tubular reabsorption of phosphate and in consequence inducing prompt phosphaturia (SLATOPOLSKY et al., 1966; ARNAUD et al., 1966). Vitamin D is not necessary for the parathyroid hormone to act on the renal tubules (ARNAUD et al., 1966). In the presence of vitamin D the infusion of parathyroid hormone causes sustained phosphaturia, since this kind of phosphaturia necessitates the mobilization of calcium and phosphate from bone, and vitamin D is necessary for physiologic concentrations of parathyroid hormone to mobilize mineral from bone (ARNAUD et al., 1966). But in the absence of vitamin D the infusion of parathyroid hormone causes only transient phosphaturia, since the lack of vitamin D prevents the mobilization of calcium and phosphate from bone (ARNAUD et al., 1966).

Thyrocalcitonin lowers plasma phosphate and induces transient phosphaturia—apparently like parathyroid hormone in the absence of vitamin D—affecting only the bone (ANAST et al., 1967). An inhibition of bone resorption leads to a fall in plasma calcium, which in consequence increases phosphate excretion (RASMUSSEN et al., 1967). The same result is obtained by simply lowering the concentration of plasma calcium, for instance, by chelating calcium with either ethylenediaminetetraacetic acid (ESTEP et al., 1965) or ethylenebis-oxyethylenenitrilotetraacetic acid (RASMUSSEN et al., 1967). The phosphaturia induced by thyrocalcitonin is not sustained, since this hormone prevents the mobilization of calcium and phosphate from bone—the similarity to the action of parathyroid hormone in the absence of vitamin D is quite impressive.

In conclusion: Parathyroid hormone induces phosphaturia and lowers plasma phosphate concentration by an effect upon renal tubular function. Thyrocalcitonin induces transient phosphaturia leading also to the lowering of plasma phosphate concentration in consequence of the fall in plasma calcium concentration brought about by the action of thyrocalcitonin upon bone. The correct adjustment of the secretion rates of both hormones brings about the relative independence in concentrations of plasma calcium and inorganic phosphate (ANAST et al., 1967).

3. Collagen Metabolism and Urinary Hydroxyproline

It is now generally agreed that the urinary excretion of hydroxyproline can be used to follow changes in the metabolism of collagen (PROCKOP and KIVIRIKKO, 1967). It is due to the unusual distribution of this hydroxyimino acid, essentially found in collagen (NEUMAN and LOGAN, 1950), and to the unique pathway of proline hydroxylation that occurs as the terminal reaction, after the complete alpha chain of protocollagen is released from the ribosomal complexes (ROSENBLOOM et al., 1967; BHATNAGAR et al., 1967). The unique pathway of hydroxyproline synthesis and the appearance of at least 95 per cent of the urinary hydroxyproline in peptide-bound form, both indicate that urinary hydroxyproline originates from the degradation of collagen.

Metabolic studies, based on a single administration of ^{14}C-proline followed by the examination of the course of the specific activity of urinary ^{14}C-hydroxyproline, suggested that most of the urinary hydroxyproline originates from the degradation of insoluble collagen, in primates about 80 per cent (AVIOLI and PROCKOP, 1967), and that only a minor part originates from the degradation of newly synthesized collagen (LINDSTEDT and PROCKOP, 1961). LAITINEN (1967) provided evidence that some of the urinary hydroxyproline originates from the recently synthesized collagen molecules that exhibit an extremely short life.

The relationship between the various forms of collagen and the urinary excretion of hydroxyproline is presented in Fig. 19. This diagram shows that the rate of hydroxyproline excretion can be affected by changes in the rates of collagen synthesis, maturation, and degradation. An increased excretion rate of urinary hydroxyproline, the most interesting sign from the clinical viewpoint, may be brought about by: an increased rate of collagen synthesis, a decreased rate of its maturation, an increased rate of its degradation, and a decreased rate of hydroxyproline metabolism to carbon dioxide and urea (PROCKOP and KIVIRIKKO, 1967).

The hydroxyproline-containing peptides from human urine include dipeptides, tripeptides (MEILMAN et al., 1963), and polypeptides of approximate molecular weight from 600 (WEISS and STEVEN, 1968) to 8,000 (HARRIS et al., 1967). The values for total hydroxyproline excreted in urine are correlated with active growth and vary in a characteristic way with age. Hence, the results of hydroxyproline excretion

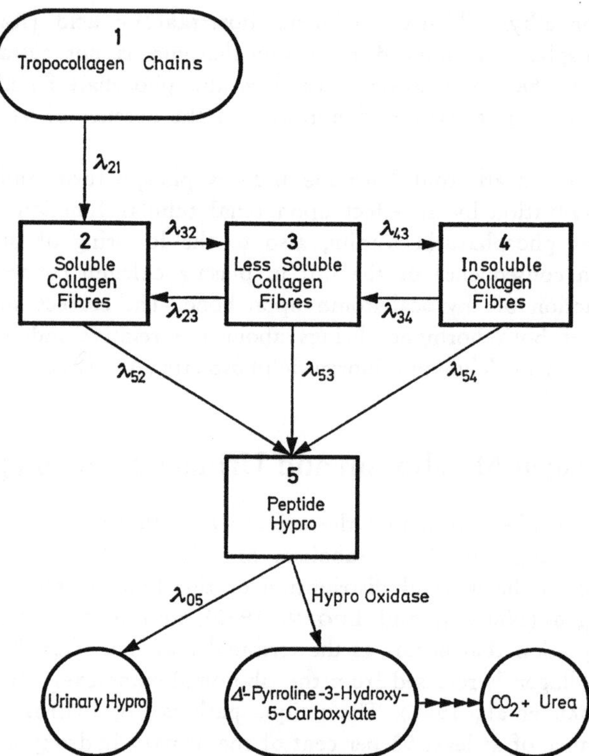

Fig. 19. Scheme of relations between collagen and urinary hydroxyproline. The fractional transfer rate constants λ_{ji} represent transfer of hydroxyproline between compartments, its excretion into urine, and degradation to carbon dioxide and urea

are expressed, either as amount per 24 hr per m^2 of body surface area (JASIN et al., 1962), or as hydroxyproline indices, that is, the micromolar ratio of hydroxyproline to creatinine with incorporated height or weight (WHARTON et al., 1967).

4. Pyrophosphate Metabolism and Urinary Pyrophosphate

In the living organism, pyrophosphate has the role of a calcification regulator. In non-mineralizing sites, it inhibits calcium phosphate precipitation and protects the connective tissue against mineralization, while, in mineralizing sites, it is destroyed by pyrophosphatase (FLEISCH and BISAZ, 1965). In addition, it seems to act as some sort of a buffer around apatite crystals, impeding both their formation and their dissolution (FLEISCH et al., 1966 b).

The normal 24-hour pyrophosphate excretion corresponds approximately to the amount of bone resorbed daily (FLEISCH and BISAZ, 1964). The parallel increments in urinary hydroxyproline and pyrophosphate in some disorders of bone metabolism (AVIOLI et al., 1965; AVIOLI et al., 1966) provide evidence that pyrophosphate excretion reflects bone resorption, and may be used as an index of this process either in parallel to or in lieu of hydroxyproline excretion.

Chapter 3

Methods of Studying Bone Mineral Metabolism

1. Plasma State and Renal Handling of Calcium and Phosphate

General Design of Study

Each patient was studied under rigidly controlled metabolic conditions in either the gynaecologic or general ward of the Institute of Oncology. A constant and controlled diet contained an average of 600 mg calcium and 900 mg phosphorus per day. After a preceding 2-day equilibration to the diet, urine samples were collected over a 24-hour period. All blood samples were taken after an overnight fast at the end of urine collection.

Preparation and Ultrafiltration of Plasma

20 ml of venous blood was obtained in well-fitting syringe, wet with heparin solution as an anticoagulant, and filled with sterile paraffin so as to exclude any contact between the blood and the air. The drawn blood was spon down under paraffin, and plasma was separated without exposure to the air (ROSE, 1957).

Anaerobic ultrafiltration was carried out on fresh plasma by the method of LAVIETES as modified by SMARSZ (1967). The Visking Nojax Casing of 3 nm pore size was used. For calcium determinations, the whole plasma and plasma ultrafiltrate were not pretreated. For phosphate determinations, 1.00 ml of whole plasma was deproteinized with 9.00 ml of 10⁰/₀ solution of trichloroacetic acid and filtered, while the plasma ultrafiltrate was not pretreated.

Preparation of Urine

After taking an appropriate volume for other determinations, urine was acidified with 1 ml of concentrated hydrochloric acid per each 100 ml of urine. For calcium determinations, 5.00 ml of the acidified urine was digested with 5 ml of concentrated nitric acid and 0.5 ml of concentrated perchloric acid, and the fairly dry residue was dissolved in water and taken into 10.0 ml volume (SZYMENDERA, 1964). For phosphate determinations, 1.00 ml of acidified urine was diluted hundredfold with distilled water.

Methods of calcium and phosphate determination (below).

Calculation of Diffusible Calcium and Phosphate

The concentrations of diffusible calcium in native plasma and plasma ultrafiltrate were assumed to be equal. No corrections were applied for plasma water or the Donnan factor for divalent cations, as in the case of divalent cations these corrections are opposite in direction and of approximately equal magnitude (cf. Chapter 2, part 1).

The concentration of plasma diffusible phosphate $[P_i]_D$ was calculated by the formula presented by WALSER (1960, 1961). The corrections for plasma water and the Donnan factor for divalent anions were applied, as in the case of divalent anions these corrections are unidirectional. The formula for plasma diffusible phosphate concentration is as follows:

$$[P_i]_D = 0.915 \cdot PW_f \cdot [P_i]_{UF} \tag{1}$$

where 0.915 is the Donnan factor for plasma phosphate, PW_f is the fractional plasma water volume equal to 0.990—0.008 [Protein], in which the concentration of protein is expressed in grams per 100 ml, and $[P_i]_{UF}$ is the concentration of inorganic phosphate in plasma ultrafiltrate.

Calculation of Renal Handling of Calcium and Phosphate

The fluid in Bowman's space is an ultrafiltrate of plasma. Since protein is an anion restricted to the blood plasma, it results in a redistribution of permeable ions according to the Donnan effect. The net result will be such that the concentration of calcium will be lower while that of phosphate will be higher in the ultrafiltrate than in the protein-free phase of plasma. Thus, in calculations of renal handling, the concentration of either ion in the plasma has to be corrected not only for protein-binding, but for the Donnan effect as well.

In practice, it is more convenient to use the concentration of either ion in the plasma ultrafiltrate, since the concentrations of either ultrafiltrable ion in plasma ultrafiltrate are in accordance with the appropriate Donnan factors. Besides, plasma ultrafiltrate has not to be corrected for the fractional plasma water content.

The calcium clearance C_{Ca}, the filtered load of calcium FL_{Ca}, the excretion of urinary calcium per unit time Ca_UV, the tubular reabsorption of calcium T_{Ca}, and further, the phosphate clearance C_P, the filtered load of phosphate FL_P, the excretion of urinary phosphate per unit time P_UV, and the tubular reabsorption of phosphate T_P—were calculated as described in the previous chapter.

2. Kinetics of Calcium Metabolism

General Design of Study

Each patient, hospitalized in the general ward of the Institute of Oncology for several days before and during the 10-day study, was not given any drugs which could have influenced the metabolism of calcium and phosphate. The patients investigated ate normal diets: their content of calcium was approximately 800—950 mg per day, and that of phosphate—900 mg per day.

Tracers

The best tracer for calcium is calcium itself, though in many studies, radio-strontium has been used as a tracer for calcium. However, strontium and calcium appear to behave indentically only as regards binding to plasma proteins (LLOYD, 1968; SZYMENDERA and MADAJEWICZ, 1968), passage from the plasma into the fluids

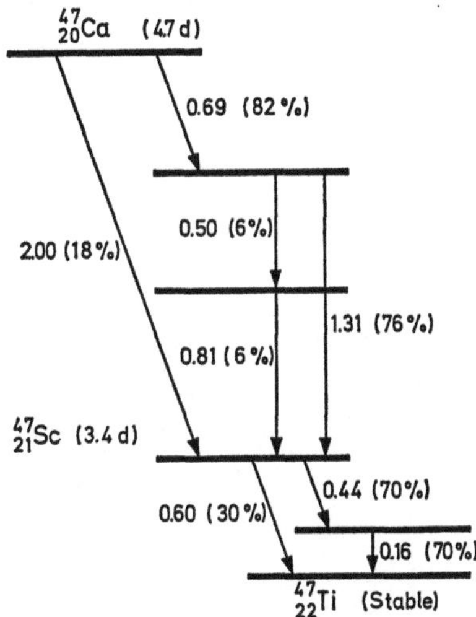

Fig. 20. The decay scheme of ^{47}Ca

of some body cavities (SAMACHSON et al., 1960), and handling by the skeleton (WASSERMAN et al., 1958; COHN et al., 1963; COHN and GUSMANO, 1967). In processes dependent upon active transport, the two elements are handled discriminatively in favour of the transport of calcium. The intestinal tract discriminates in favour of the transport of calcium (WASSERMAN et al., 1958; WASSERMAN, 1960; DELLA ROSA et al., 1965; SAMACHSON, 1966; SPENCER et al., 1966; HART and SPENCER, 1967). The secretion of calcium is favoured also by the salivary (SAMACHSON et al., 1965) and the mammary glands (WASSERMAN et al., 1958; LOUGH et al., 1960). On the other hand, the kidneys apparently discriminate in favour of the secretion of strontium (WASSERMAN et al., 1958; COHN et al., 1963; SPENCER et al., 1966). But, since there is no difference between the filtered loads of calcium and strontium (SZYMENDERA and MADAJEWICZ, 1968), and since only the reabsorption of calcium from all parts of the nephron is an active process (LASSITER et al., 1963), the discrimination against strontium reabsorption seems to be responsible for the greater excretion of strontium in urine. Hence, the metabolically active membranes differentiate in the same way between calcium and strontium. The elimination of this discriminative property in intestinal segments by metabolic inhibitors (WASSERMAN, 1960) provides further evidence that the active transport of strontium differs significantly from that of calcium.

Owing to this discrimination, for studying the kinetics of calcium only the radio-isotopes of calcium were used: ^{45}Ca and ^{47}Ca. The former nuclide, a soft beta-emitter of 0.254 MeV electrons, is convenient when balance studies are being made and calcium is being isolated from excreta. The long half-life of 165 days is the only disadvantage of this isotope for clinical research, since the heavy body burden imposed by the administration of higher activity limits its use. The latter nuclide, an emitter of gamma rays, is more convenient, since the measurements of the tracer in samples, in entire collections of excreta, and in whole body are extremely easy. The short half-life of 4.7 days is the only disadvantage of this isotope, preventing long-lasting

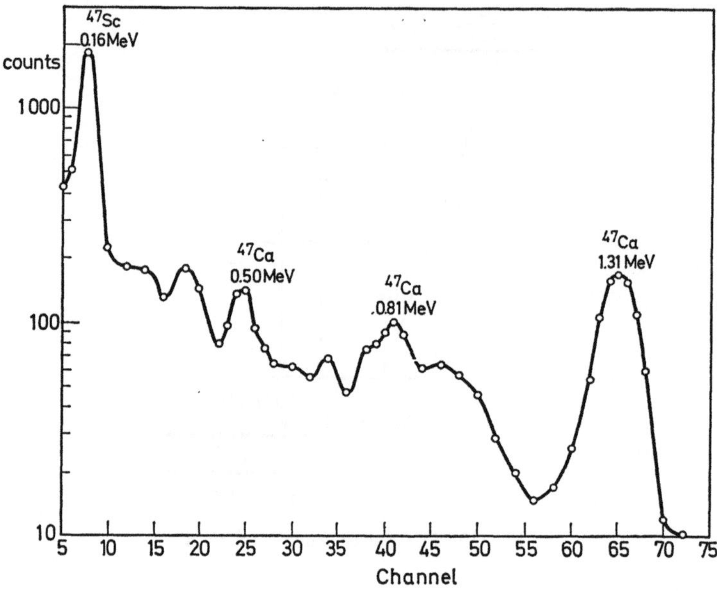

Fig. 21. Gamma ray spectrum of ^{47}Ca and ^{47}Sc measured with 2 in. diameter and 1.5 in. thick NaI(Tl) crystal and pulse-height analyser

investigations. The decay scheme of ^{47}Ca and its spectrum are presented in Figs. 20 and 21.

Kinetic Study

Each study began early in the morning with rapid injection into an antecubital vein of radiocalcium dissolved in sterile isotonic saline (supplied by The Radiochemical Centre, Amersham, England). The dose of tracer did not exceed either 1 μCi ^{47}Ca or 0.3 μCi ^{45}Ca per kg of body weight. Blood samples were taken from the opposite antecubital vein for radioactivity and calcium assays at 30 min and at 1, 2, 4, 6, 8, 24, 36 and 48 hours following injection, and then daily for the next 5 to 7 days. In patients given ^{45}Ca, spot urine collections were made at 71—73, 95—97, 119—121, 143—145, and 167—169 hours following the injection; the specific activity of each spot urine sample was taken as corresponding to that of plasma at the midpoint of the interval (SZYMENDERA et al., 1967 a).

In patients given ^{47}Ca, urine was collected in 24-hr pooled specimens; while in those given ^{45}Ca, urine was collected at 24-hr intervals till the third day, when both spot collections and 22-hr collections were begun. Faecal specimens were collected daily for about 9 days after the isotope injection. A brilliant blue marker or carmine red marker was given orally at the time of the last blood collection or the last spot urine voiding, and faeces collected before the passage of the faecal marker were included in the study.

Preparation of Samples for Analysis and Radioactivity Determinations

The ^{47}Ca radioactivity in the plasma, acidified urine, and homogenized faeces was measured at constant geometry on 20.0 ml samples. All assays were carried out with a scintillation detector with a NaI(Tl) crystal and pulse height analyzer (SC-78, Tracerlab) calibrated to discriminate against radiation from the ^{47}Sc daughter of ^{47}Ca (Figs. 20 and 21). A fraction of the injected dose of ^{47}Ca was simultaneously assayed as a standard.

The ^{45}Ca radioactivity was measured in samples of equal area and density. For preparing identical samples for counting, a fraction of the injected dose of ^{45}Ca taken as a standard was not pretreated, the plasma was deproteinized with trichloroacetic acid and the filtrate was used, urine was mineralized with nitric and perchloric acid and taken to a known volume, stool was homogenized and ashed with nitric and perchloric acid and taken to a known volume. The counting samples were prepared in the following steps: a volume with a strictly known amount of calcium was (a) made up to a standard weight of 4.1 mg calcium; (b) precipitated as calcium oxalate; (c) plated by filtering onto filter paper disk of 20 mm in diameter; (d) attached to an aluminium planchette and dried (SZYMENDERA et al., 1967 a). The sample were measured with a monomol end-window gas-flow proportional counter (FD-1, Tracerlab) and an automatic sample changer (SC-6D, Tracerlab). The counting geometry was identical for both the standards and unknowns. The counting error in either technique did not exceed 1 per cent.

Preliminary Presentation of Data

Stable calcium was measured in relevant samples of plasma, urine, and faeces (see below). The activity of the measured material corrected for physical decay was expressed as a percentage of the dose of injected radiocalcium. The plasma and spot urine activities were further expressed as the specific activity values, that is, as percentage of dose per gram calcium, and from these the curve in Fig. 22 was constructed.

The activity recovered in excreta, expressed as percentage of dose per 24-hour urine collection and daily stool specimens, was further expressed as the cumulative excretion in urine and faeces, from which the curves presented in Fig. 23 were constructed.

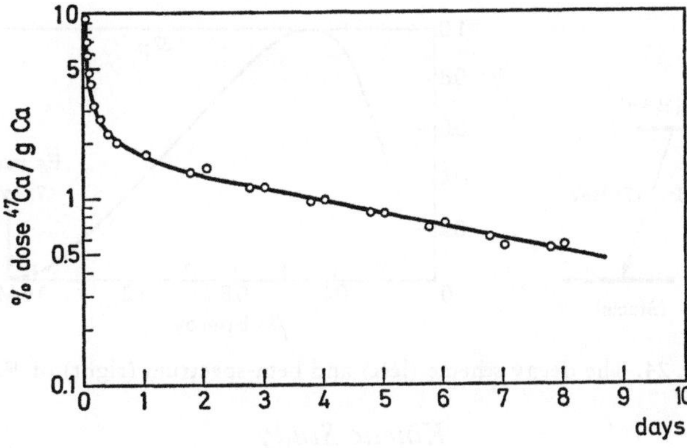

Fig. 22. A semilogarithmic plot of plasma and spot urine calcium specific activity against days (case Z.A.)

3*

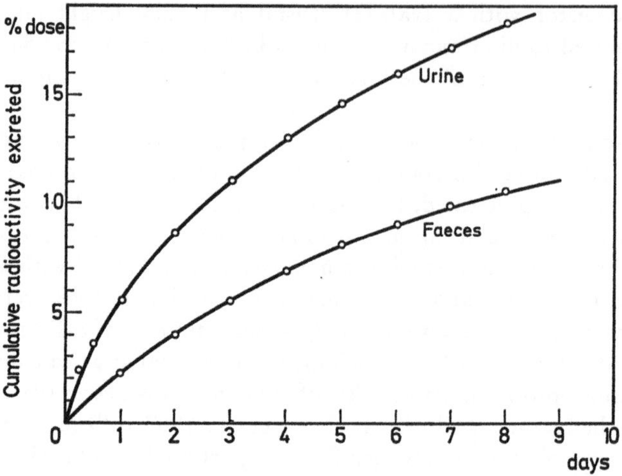

Fig. 23. Cumulative excretions of radiocalcium in urine and faeces plotted against days (same case)

3. Kinetics of Inorganic Phosphate Metabolism

General Design of Study

Each patient, hospitalized in the general ward of the Institute of Oncology for several days before and during the 10-day study, was not given any drugs which could have influenced calcium and phosphate metabolism. The patients ate normal diets: their phosphate content was approximately 900 mg per day.

Tracer

Only ^{32}P was used as a tracer. This nuclide is a hard beta-emitter of 1.71 MeV electrons, and has a convenient half-life of 14.3 days. Owing to the relatively high energy of its electrons and therefore its low self-absorption, it is convenient for preparing samples of equal density. The decay scheme of ^{32}P and its spectrum are presented in Fig. 24.

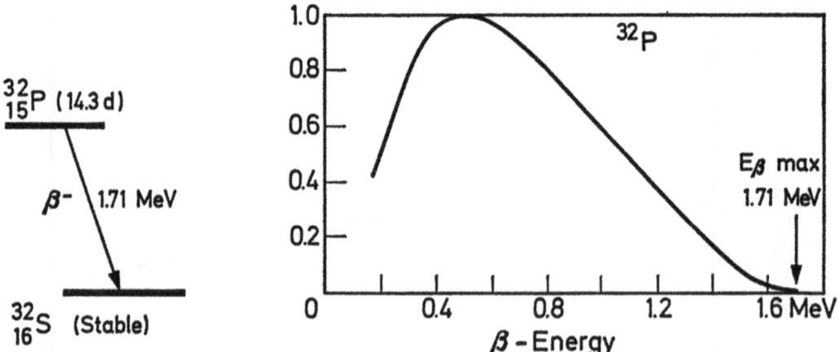

Fig. 24. The decay scheme (left) and beta-spectrum (right) of ^{32}P

Kinetic Study

Each study began early in the morning with rapid injection into an antecubital vein of carrier-free radiophosphate dissolved in sterile isotonic saline (supplied by

The Radiochemical Centre, Amersham, England). The dose of tracer did not exceed 0.6 µCi per kg of body weight. Blood samples were taken from the opposite antecubital vein for radioactivity and phosphate assays at 1, 2.5, 4, 6, 10, 24, and 34 hours following injection, and then spot urine collections were made at 48—50, 72—74, 96—98, 120—122, 144—146, 168—170, and 192—194 hours following the injection; the specific activity of each spot urine sample was taken as corresponding to that of plasma at the midpoint of the interval.

Urine was collected in 2-liter polythene containers. Voidings were pooled in 24-hour specimens till the third day following the isotope injection, when both spot and 22-hour collections were begun. Faecal specimens were collected daily for about 10 days after the isotope injection. A carmine red marker was given orally at the time of the last spot urine voiding, and faeces collected before the passage of the faecal marker were included in the study.

Preparation of Samples for Analysis and Radioactivity Determination

The ^{32}P radioactivity was measured in samples of equal area and density. Identical samples for counting were prepared as follows: (a) the dose of ^{32}P was diluted with Na_2HPO_4 (25 mg P per 100 ml solution) to obtain 0.5 per cent dose ^{32}P per 100 ml solution; (b) 2.00 ml of plasma was deproteinized with 18.00 ml of 5 per cent solution of trichloroacetic acid and filtered; (c) spot urine and pooled urine were acidified (1 ml of concentrated hydrochloric acid per 100 ml urine) and filtered; (d) 50.0 ml of pooled urine was boiled for 30 minutes to hydrolyze the organic compounds of phosphate, cooled, and then made up to the initial 50.0 ml volume; (e) 5—10 g of homogenized faeces was weighed in a Kjeldahl flask, ashed with nitric and perchloric acid, and taken into 25.0 ml volume.

The counting samples were prepared in the following steps: (a) volumes containing 2.5 ± 0.05 mg P were taken: 10.0 ml of standard equal to 0.05 per cent dose; appropriate volumes of spot urine, hydrolyzed urine, and faecal ash (if necessary, these samples were made up to 10 ml volume); 10.0 ml of plasma filtrate to which 2.5 mg of P (as Na_2HPO_4) was added; (b) to each sample in a 50 ml Jena glass, 2 ml of magnesium citrate mixture of Fiske (MATHISON, 1909), and 4 ml of concentrated ammonia water (sp. gr. 0.90) were added; (c) the glass was closed with a rubber-stopper and shaken for 10 minutes and then allowed to stand at least 2 hours (PETERS and VAN SLYKE, 1961); (d) the $NH_4MgPO_4 \cdot 6\,H_2O$ crystalline precipitate was plated by filtering onto filter paper disk of 20 mm diameter, attached to an aluminium planchette, and dried.

The samples were measured with a mica (1.36 mg per cm²) end-window Geiger tube (BAT-25) mounted in an automatic sample changer (SC-6D, Tracerlab) and connected to a timing scaler (SC-83, Tracerlab). The counting geometry was identical for both the standards and unknowns. The counting error did not exceed 2 per cent.

Preliminary Presentation of Data

Stable inorganic phosphate was measured in relevant samples of plasma, urine, and faeces (see below). The activity of the measured material corrected for physical decay was expressed as a percentage of the dose of injected radiophosphate. The plasma and spot urine activities were further expressed as the specific activity values, that is, as percentage of dose per gram phosphorus, from which the curve presented in Fig. 25 was constructed.

The activity recovered in excreta, expressed as percentage of dose per 24-hour urine collections and daily stool specimens, was further expressed as the cumulative excretion in urine and faeces, from which the curves presented in Fig. 26 were constructed.

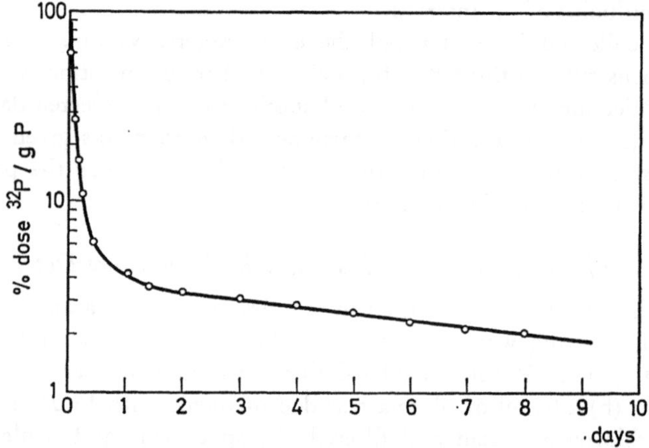

Fig. 25. A semilogarithmic plot of plasma and spot urine inorganic phosphate specific activity against days (case Z.K.)

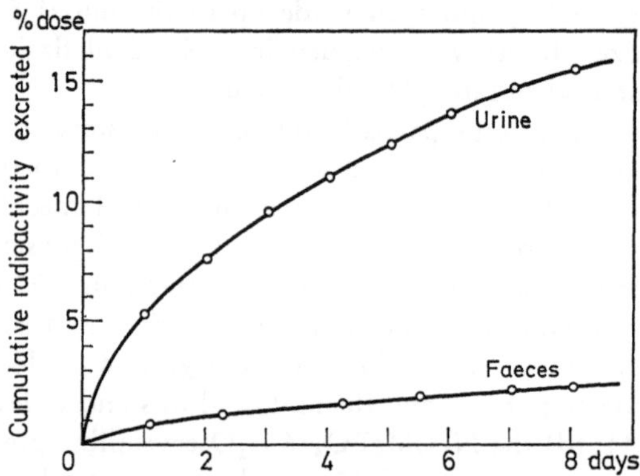

Fig. 26. Cumulative excretions of radiophosphate in urine and faeces plotted against days (same case)

4. Multicompartmental Analysis of Calcium and Phosphate Kinetics

Calcium and phosphate data were analyzed in terms of a compartmental model. Two arbitrary assumptions concerning the model were made. First, that the systems of exchangeable calcium and inorganic phosphate are in steady states, which is physiologically reasonable, since the studies were done after equilibration to a constant regimen. Second, that the systems of exchangeable calcium and phosphate are compartmentalized, which is consistent with the data.

All data of either the calcium or phosphate kinetic study, from 30 minutes till 7—8 days of the study, were satisfied with a sum of three exponentials, extracted by the "peeling" technique. Thus, three exchanging compartments in each system were proposed. To analyze the data, an open three-compartment mammillary system model was chosen, as presented in Fig. 27.

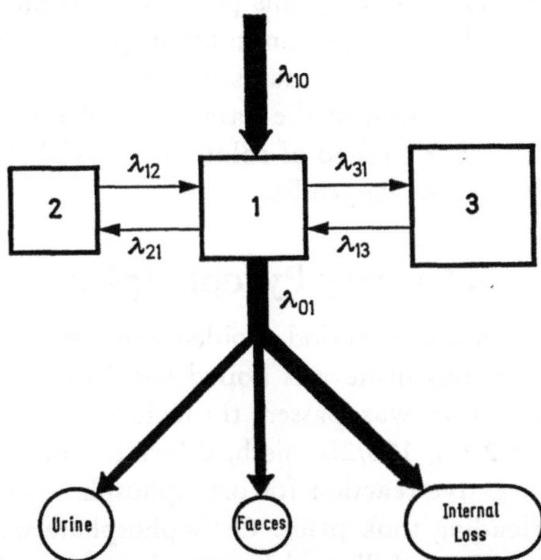

Fig. 27. Compartmental model of calcium and inorganic phosphate metabolism compatible with a three-exponential plasma activity disappearance curve. The pool of either ion is in isotopic equilibrium within 15—20 minutes in Compartment 1, within a few hours in Compartment 2, and within two days in Compartment 3. λ_{ij} represents the intercompartmental fractional transfer rate into compartment i from compartment j; λ_{10} is the fractional rate of entry of either ion into Compartment 1 from areas outside the exchangeable pool; λ_{01} is the fractional rate of loss of either ion from the exchangeable pool, and includes the excretion into urine and faeces and internal loss, into bone in the case of calcium, and into bone and forming organic compounds in the case of phosphate

Urinary and faecal calcium and phosphate are assumed to come directly from the central compartment, and also both ions absorbed from the diet are assumed to enter the central compartment, which is physiologically reasonable. Urinary and faecal radioactivities do not account for all the radiocalcium and, to an even greater degree, radiophosphate lost from the system. The difference between the turnover rate of the exchangeable pool and the excretion rate into urine and faeces represents the internal loss: to nonexchanging bone in the case of calcium, and both to nonexchanging bone and to forming organic compounds of long half-life in the case of phosphate. There are no criteria for choosing the exact compartment as the site of the internal loss, but since blood is the central exchanger for the whole body, it seemed reasonable to assume the central compartment, of which the blood is a part, as the site of this loss. Calcium and phosphate returning to the exchangeable pool from nonexchanging bone and from the breakdown of organic compounds are both assumed to enter the central compartment, too.

The notation for parameters of the model followed that of BROWNELL et al. (1968): $M_i =$ grams of calcium or phosphorus in compartment i of the exchangeable calcium or phosphate system; $\lambda_{ij} =$ fractional rate of calcium or phosphorus transfer into compartment i from compartment j in units of days^{-1}; $\varrho_{ij} = \lambda_{ij} M_j =$ amount of calcium or phosphorus transferred into compartment i from compartment j in grams per day; ϱ_{i0} = amount of calcium or phosphorus transferred into compartment i from areas outside the exchangeable pool in grams per day; ϱ_{0i} = amount of calcium or phosphorus excreted from compartment i in grams per day.

For certain ϱ_{ij} of calcium the notation of AUBERT and MILHAUD (1960) was used: V_u = calcium excreted in the urine in grams per day; V_f = endogenous faecal calcium in grams per day; V_F = total faecal calcium in grams per day; V_0^+ = calcium deposited internally (accreted) in forming bone in grams per day.

The formulae for determination of the parameters of this model have been given by LEVALLEN et al. (1959). The method of solution, a trivial elimination method, and the formulae are presented in the Appendix.

5. Urinary Pyrophosphate

During the 24-hour collection period, voided urine was pooled in a cooled jar. A homogeneous sample of this urine was boiled for 2 minutes to destroy the pyrophosphatase. 4.00 ml of urine was passed through a column 11 mm in diameter, containing 10 ml Dowex 2×8, 100/200 mesh, chloride form. The column was rinsed with 20 ml water; the negative reaction for orthophosphate of the rinsing eluate was indicative that no overloading took place. Orthophosphate was initially eluted with 100 ml of 0.14 N KCl, pH 5.0, followed by 20 ml water, and the remaining pyrophosphate was then eluted with 50 ml of 0.5 N HCl. The elution pattern of urinary ortho- and pyrophosphate is shown in Fig. 28. This procedure is a modification of the methods of FLEISCH et al. (1964) and AVIOLI et al. (1965). After hydrolyzing the pyrophosphate for 30 minutes in a boiling-water bath, phosphorus was estimated by the method of CHEN et al. (1956).

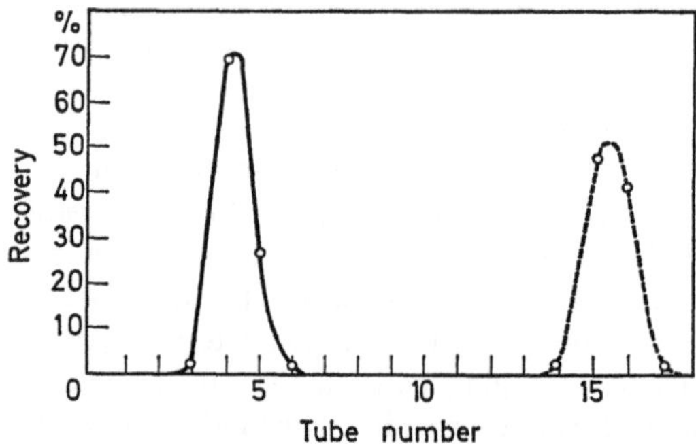

Fig. 28. Elution recovery pattern of 250 μg of ortho- and 2.5 μg of pyrophosphate. Ordinate represents the recovery percentage, abscissa the successive 10 ml volumes of eluate, each in a separate tube. Tube 1 represents the column hold up volume, tubes 2—11 the KCl elutions containing orthophosphate, tubes 12—13 the distilled water washings, tubes 14—18 the HCl elutions of pyrophosphate

6. Other Methods

Calcium was titrated with disodium dihydrogen ethylenediamine tetraacetate (EDTA), using calcein (Sigma) as an indicator and ultraviolet-light illumination (BETT and FRASER, 1959). Standard procedure was applied for plasma and ultrafiltrate calcium. Owing to interference from the high phosphate concentrations normally found in the urine, 0.1 M solution of sodium citrate was added prior to titration (McPherson, 1965). Owing to interference from both the high concentrations of phosphate and the presence of iron, manganese, and other metals in faecal ash, 1 per cent solution of sodium cyanide was additionally added prior to titration (McPherson, 1965).

Inorganic phosphate was measured in deproteinized plasma, in plasma ultrafiltrate, in diluted urine and faecal ash by the method of Gomori (1942). Plasma alkaline phosphatase was determined by the method of King and Armstrong (1956). Creatinine in plasma and urine was determined by the method of Taussky (1961).

The statistical analyses were performed according to methods given by Snedecor (1956).

The Metabolism of Bone Mineral in Malignancy without Evidence of Bone Destruction

Most patients with malignant disease exhibit normal metabolism of bone mineral, various disturbances in it being found in only a small number. Among the disturbances found, hypercalcaemia has long been the most frequently, and regularly reported phenomenon. In the last decade, owing to a remarkable increase in interest in calcium and phosphate metabolism, hypercalcaemia has been observed in patients with a wide variety of cancers, chiefly with bone metastases, but without overt bone metastases as well. MYERS (1960) found hypercalcaemia in 430 patients from a 5-year group of patients with malignant tumours. Of these patients, 225 (52.3 per cent) had cancer of the breast, 33 (7.7 per cent)—lymphomas, 29 (6.7 per cent)—cancer of the lung, 18 (4.2 per cent)—cancer of the kidney, 12 (2.8 per cent)—cancer of the uterine cervix, 11 (2.5 per cent)—plasmacytoma, and the remaining 102 (23.8 per cent) had miscellaneous tumours. Roentgenograms of the skeleton were negative for metastases in 56 (13.0 per cent) patients from this group.

Hypercalcaemia occurs in about 10 per cent of patients with radiological evidence of widespread destruction of bone by metastases (WOODARD, 1953). Of course, the roentgenographic diagnosis of metastatic cancer is often unsatisfactory in widespread but small lesions. This has been proved by post-mortem examinations, which demonstrated that about 85 per cent of patients dying of the tumours which commonly metastasize to bone had bone secondaries, though in many cases they were not visualized by roentgenography (JAFFE, 1958). Recently, bone scanning with radioactive strontium that is deposited in the vicinity of bone metastasis (CHARKES et al., 1966) has increased the percentage of detected bone secondaries (CHARKES et al., 1966; McCREADY et al., 1966; SKLAROFF and CHARKES, 1967 a; SKLAROFF and CHARKES, 1967 b; SPENCER et al., 1967). Thus, the destruction of bone by metastases explains hypercalcaemia in some patients with tumours.

There remain a good many patients with hypercalcaemia in the absence of bone metastases, which is produced by different mechanism. PLIMPTON and GELLHORN (1956) suggested, and MYERS et al. (1966) produced supporting evidence that the primary defect in hypercalcaemia of cancer is an enhanced resorption of bone, which exceeds the accretion rate which is also increased. But the mechanism of this enhanced resorption may differ.

Some tumours produce a parathyroid-like substance. An ectopic elaboration of parathyroid hormone by cancers accounts for the chemical syndrome of hypercalcaemia and hypophosphataemia. Such a substance had been isolated in tumour extracts from hypercalcaemic patients with carcinoma of the kidney or the lung

(TASHJIAN et al., 1964; SHERWOOD et al., 1967). In a significant percentage of patients with bronchogenic carcinoma there were found higher than normal concentrations of parathyroid hormone in plasma (BERSON and YALOW, 1966).

Other tumours may produce osteolytic sterols. The osteolytic action of this sterol accounts for the chemical syndrome of hypercalcaemia not associated with hypophosphataemia but accompanied by normal or even slightly elevated concentrations of plasma phosphate. This syndrome is chiefly associated with breast cancer (THOMAS et al., 1960). The osteolytic sterol was found in 11 of the 12 human breast cancers removed at operation, and appeared to be chemically close to vitamin D: Δ7-sitosterol acetate and sigmasteryl acetate (GORDAN et al., 1966; GORDAN, 1967).

It seems possible to distinguish, on the basis of the elegant series of investigations, another very interesting clinical entity. Ten years ago medullary carcinoma of the thyroid gland was first described by HAZARD et al. (1959). This variety of thyroid carcinoma formed 6.5 per cent (57 out of 885 patients) of thyroid carcinomas diagnosed and treated at the Mayo Clinic (WOOLNER et al., 1961). WILLIAMS et al. (1966) suggested the origin of medullary carcinoma from the parafollicular (clear, C) cells, and MEYER and ABDEL-BARI (1968) demonstrated thyrocalcitonin-like activity in this variety of cancer. CUNLIFFE et al. (1968) detected a great excess of calcitonin in plasma and a 5,000-fold excess of calcitonin in tumour tissue, and RINIKER et al. (1968) and NEHER et al. (1968) isolated from the tumour tissue two highly active calcitonin peptides characterized as calcitonin M, a peptide with 32 amino acids, and calcitonin D, a dimer of M.

In patients with C-cell cancer a tendency toward hypocalcaemia might be anticipated. But, either the parathyroid glands compensate functionally for the effect of excessive thyrocalcitonin (MEYER and ABDEL-BARI, 1968; CUNLIFFE et al., 1968), or bone may become refractory to thyrocalcitonin (MEYER and ABDEL-BARI); one way or the other, hypocalcaemia is a rare phenomenon. Nevertheless, greater attention should be paid to hypocalcaemia in malignancy.

The bulk of studies upon bone mineral disturbances associated with cancer concerned only the plasma concentrations of total calcium and inorganic phosphate, and the urinary excretion of both elements. There have been only a few reports on the plasma state of calcium and inorganic phosphate, their renal handling, and their kinetics. The present chapter has been designed to further the study of calcium and inorganic phosphate metabolism in patients without apparent bone destruction, also the influence of X-ray castration, which is a side-effect of combined curie- and X-ray therapy of carcinoma of the uterine cervix.

1. Metabolism of Calcium and Inorganic Phosphate

1.1. Clinical Material

All patients were classified in three groups, arranged according to whether (1) the plasma state and renal handling of calcium and phosphate, (2) the kinetics of calcium, or (3) the kinetics of inorganic phosphate were studied.

The first group (patients No. 1—32) includes: 27 patients with carcinoma of the uterine cervix, two with mesothelioma of the peritoneum, two with carcinoma of the ovary, and one with dysgerminoma of the ovary. The second group (patients No. 33

to 48) includes: 6 patients with carcinoma of the skin, six with carcinoma of the lip, two with carcinoma of the larynx, and two with other cancers. The third group (patients No. 49—55) includes: 2 patients with mesothelioma of the pulmonum, two with cancer of the skin, two with primary polycythaemia, and one with carcinoma of the larynx. The diagnoses are given in Table 1.

Table 1. *Clinical data*

Patient	Sex	Age (years)	Diagnosis
1-M.B.	F	39	Carcinoma of the uterine cervix, st. 0
2-W.M.	F	28	Carcinoma of the uterine cervix, st. 0
3-M.L.	F	48	Carcinoma of the uterine cervix, st. 0
4-Z.S.	F	42	Carcinoma of the uterine cervix, st. I
5-M.K.	F	30	Carcinoma of the uterine cervix, st. I
6-K.A.	F	34	Carcinoma of the uterine cervix, st. I
7-A.S.	F	44	Carcinoma of the uterine cervix, st. I
8-E.J.	F	35	Carcinoma of the uterine cervix, st. I
9-J.K	F	45	Carcinoma of the uterine cervix, st. I
10-J.C.	F	47	Carcinoma of the uterine cervix, st. I
11-H.G.	F	27	Carcinoma of the uterine cervix, st. I
12-M.N.	F	42	Carcinoma of the uterine cervix, st. I
13-I.S.	F	43	Carcinoma of the uterine cervix, st. I
14-B.G.	F	37	Carcinoma of the uterine cervix, st. I
15-W.K.	F	43	Carcinoma of the uterine cervix, st. II
16-B.K.	F	43	Carcinoma of the uterine cervix, st. II
17-D.K.	F	37	Carcinoma of the uterine cervix, st. II
18-S.W.	F	42	Carcinoma of the uterine cervix, st. II
19-Z.G.	F	50	Carcinoma of the uterine cervix, st. II
20-H.P.	F	39	Carcinoma of the uterine cervix, st. II
21-W.O.	F	34	Carcinoma of the uterine cervix, st. II
22-T.S.	F	33	Carcinoma of the uterine cervix, st. II
23-H.B.	F	42	Carcinoma of the uterine cervix, st. II
24-E.D.	F	43	Carcinoma of the uterine cervix, st. III
25-M.G.	F	46	Carcinoma of the uterine cervix, st. III
26-Z.S.	F	44	Carcinoma of the uterine cervix, st. III
27-S.D.	F	44	Carcinoma of the uterine cervix, st. III
28-K.C.	F	40	Mesothelioma of the peritoneum
29-J.S.	F	20	Mesothelioma of the peritoneum
30-W.B.	F	27	Cancer of the ovary, after right oophorectomy
31-J.K.	F	38	Cancer of the ovary
32-E.G.	F	25	Dysgerminoma of the ovary
33-T.J.	F	60	Cancer of the skin
34-T.J.	F	54	Cancer of the skin
35-K.S.	F	58	Cancer of the skin
36-P.M.	F	46	Cancer of the skin
37-P.S.	M	67	Cancer of the skin
38-B.J.	M	55	Cancer of the skin
39-S.F.	M	45	Cancer of the lip
40-W.J.	M	46	Cancer of the lip
41-Z.A.	M	55	Cancer of the lip
42-M.S.	M	49	Cancer of the lip
43-W.H	M	28	Cancer of the lip
44-P.B.	M	56	Cancer of the lip
45-O.S.	M	40	Tumour of the neck
46-Z.W.	M	30	Cancer of the larynx

Patient	Sex	Age (years)	Diagnosis
47-G.S.	M	36	Synovioma of the knee joint
48-G.W.	M	67	Cancer of the larynx
49-W.D.	M	50	Primary polycythaemia
50-K.D.	F	48	Primary polycythaemia
51-P.J.	M	56	Cancer of the larynx
52-J.A.	M	46	Mesothelioma of the lung
53-J.M.	F	52	Mesothelioma of the lung
54-S.R.	M	56	Cancer of the skin
55-A.M.	M	64	Cancer of the skin

1.2. Results

Plasma State of Calcium and Inorganic Phosphate

Observed data for the first group of patients are given in Table 2. The mean pyrophosphate excretion in 16 normal subjects (AVIOLI and HENNEMAN, 1966), and the mean values of remaining parameters in 25 normal subjects (SMARSZ, in press) have been also included. The group has been divided into four subgroups representing the various stages of cervical cancer, and a fifth subgroup including the remaining cancers. Since the analysis of variance of each parameter showed no significant difference between the subgroup means, the group has been treated as a single sample.

The concentration of plasma protein, 6.6 ± 0.13 g/100 ml (mean $\pm$ SE), was significantly lower than the normal mean 7.5 ± 0.15 g/100 ml ($p < 0.01$). In seven of the 32 patients the concentration of plasma protein was below the inferior limit of the normal range. The level of plasma alkaline phosphatase slightly exceeded the upper limit of the normal range in three of the 32 patients, and was within the normal range in the remainder. The mean level of plasma alkaline phosphatase, 10.3 ± 0.59 King-Armstrong units/100 ml, was not significantly different from the normal mean 9.5 ± 0.53 K-A units/100 ml. Although in all patients the excretion of urinary inorganic pyrophosphate was within the normal range, the mean 2.6 ± 0.22 mg/day differed significantly from the normal mean 4.0 ± 0.45 mg/day ($p < 0.01$). Both indices of bone dynamics militate against an enhanced bone resorption.

The plasma concentration of total calcium, 8.99 ± 0.116 mg/100 ml, was lower than the normal mean 9.58 ± 0.076 mg/100 ml, and the variability in total calcium concentration of this group was greater than that of the normal subjects ($p < 0.001$). Only in one patient with cancer of the ovary (case 31-J.K.) did the concentration of total plasma calcium exceed the upper limit, while in as many as 13 patients the concentration was below the inferior limit of the normal range. The plasma concentration of diffusible calcium, 5.38 ± 0.070 mg/100 ml, was significantly lower than the normal mean 5.70 ± 0.072 mg/100 ml ($p < 0.01$). Only in one patient with cancer of the uterine cervix stage III (case 26-Z.S.) did the concentration slightly exceed the upper limit of the normal range, due to lowered protein-binding of calcium, while in as many as 14 patients the concentration of diffusible calcium was below the inferior limit of the normal range. In ten of these 14 patients, this was due to the lowered concentration of total calcium, and in the remaining 4 patients, this was due to high protein-binding of calcium.

Table 2. *Indices of bone dynamics and plasma state of calcium and inorganic phosphate*

Patient	Plasma Protein	Alk. P'tase	Urinary PP_i	$[Ca]_P$	$[Ca]_D$	Ca_{PB}		K_{CaProt}	$[P_i]_P$	$[P_i]_D$	P_{PB}
	g/100 ml	K-A U	mg/day	mg/100 ml		%	mg/g protein	M	mg/100 ml		%
1-M.B.	6.6	8.0	1.7	8.77	5.48	37.5	0.50	0.0120	3.12	2.85	8.5
2-W.M.	7.8	12.1	3.0	9.27	5.50	40.7	0.48	0.0125	2.80	2.21	21.2
3-M.L.	6.2	10.7	2.2	9.13	5.45	40.3	0.59	0.0098	2.90	2.58	11.0
Group mean	6.9	10.3	2.3	9.06	5.48	39.2	0.52	0.0114	2.94	2.55	13.6
±SE	±0.48	±1.20	±0.38	±0.149	±0.015	±1.01	±0.034	±0.00083	±0.095	±0.185	±0.42
4-Z.S.	6.6	17.9	1.3	9.23	5.73	37.9	0.53	0.0118	2.73	2.34	14.3
5-M.K.	6.3	10.6	3.5	8.69	4.33	50.2	0.69	0.0065	3.36	2.89	14.0
6-K.A.	6.0	9.1	3.4	9.02	6.01	33.4	0.50	0.0131	2.67	2.30	13.8
7-A.S.	6.9	10.8	4.8	9.61	5.75	40.2	0.56	0.0111	4.38	3.91	10.7
8-E.J.	6.8	7.2	2.4	8.87	5.55	37.4	0.49	0.0125	3.33	2.87	13.8
9-J.K.	7.2	12.2	2.3	8.65	5.18	40.1	0.48	0.0118	3.60	3.07	14.7
10-J.C.	7.2	7.0	1.9	9.07	5.16	43.1	0.54	0.0103	3.80	3.24	14.7
11-H.G.	6.4	6.4	2.1	9.32	5.61	39.8	0.58	0.0104	3.30	2.84	14.1
12-M.N.	5.9	5.8	4.0	9.23	5.00	45.8	0.72	0.0073	2.30	1.98	13.7
13-I.S.	7.9	8.8	3.0	9.97	5.80	41.8	0.53	0.0120	3.81	3.39	11.0
14-B.G.	5.6	9.5	1.3	8.38	5.47	34.7	0.52	0.0115	3.00	2.59	13.5
Group mean	6.6	9.6	2.7	9.09	5.42	40.4	0.56	0.0108	3.30	2.86	13.5
±SE	±0.20	±1.03	±0.34	±0.136	±0.143	±1.45	±0.024	±0.00063	±0.180	±0.165	±0.41
15-W.K.	6.0	12.2	2.0	9.35	5.00	46.5	0.73	0.0072	3.60	3.10	13.8
16-B.K.	5.8	16.8	2.3	8.71	5.32	38.9	0.58	0.0098	3.20	2.68	16.3
17-D.K.	7.1	10.9	2.2	8.13	5.38	33.8	0.39	0.0156	3.31	2.51	24.2

PP_i = inorganic pyrophosphate; $[Ca]_P$ = plasma total calcium concentration; $[Ca]_D$ = plasma diffusible calcium concentration; Ca_{PB} = plasma protein-bound calcium; K_{CaProt} = dissociation constant of calcium proteinate; $[P_i]_P$ = plasma total inorganic phosphate concentration; $[P_i]_D$ = plasma diffusible inorganic phosphate concentration; P_{PB} = plasma protein-bound inorganic phosphate; F = ratio of the between-subgroups variance estimate to the within-subgroups variance estimate; p = probability that the means or variances for all patients and normal subjects are not different—values higher than 0.05 are nonsignificant (NS).

Table 2 (continued)

Patient	Plasma Protein	Alk. P'tase	Urinary PP_i	$[Ca]_P$	$[Ca]_D$	Ca_{PB}		K_{CaProt}	$[P_i]_P$	$[P_i]_D$	P_{PB}
	g/100 ml	K-A U	mg/day	mg/100 ml		%	mg/g protein	M	mg/100 ml		%
18-S.W.	6.4	7.0	1.6	8.46	5.08	40.0	0.53	0.0105	2.90	2.58	11.1
19-Z.G.	6.2	11.6	1.8	8.26	4.57	44.7	0.60	0.0082	2.93	2.52	14.0
20-H.P.	6.2	7.5	2.1	8.71	5.50	36.9	0.52	0.0116	2.54	2.10	17.4
21-W.O.	6.7	8.3	6.1	8.64	5.16	40.3	0.52	0.0108	3.16	2.71	14.4
22-T.S.	6.0	11.1	3.6	9.03	5.63	37.7	0.57	0.0107	3.20	2.59	19.2
23-H.B.	6.7	14.2	2.8	9.03	5.32	41.1	0.55	0.0102	3.02	2.59	14.4
Group mean	6.3	11.1	2.7	8.70	5.22	40.0	0.55	0.0105	3.10	2.60	16.1
±SE	±0.14	±1.06	±0.47	±0.130	±0.105	±1.29	±0.030	±0.00078	±0.099	±0.086	±1.28
24-E.D.	5.4	15.0	1.3	8.26	5.32	35.6	0.54	0.0106	3.40	3.03	10.8
25-M.G	5.5	8.9	3.1	9.06	5.55	38.8	0.64	0.0092	2.57	2.40	6.7
26-Z.S.	7.5	9.5	2.7	9.52	6.17	35.2	0.45	0.0153	2.73	2.32	14.9
27-S.D.	5.8	9.6	1.5	9.03	5.65	37.4	0.58	0.0104	2.83	2.53	10.6
Group mean	6.1	10.8	2.2	8.97	5.67	36.8	0.55	0.0114	2.88	2.57	10.8
±SE	±0.49	±1.43	±0.44	±0.261	±0.180	±0.83	±0.040	±0.00135	±0.181	±0.159	±1.67
28-K.C.	6.4	14.1	1.4	7.67	4.79	37.5	0.45	0.0118	2.77	2.38	14.1
29-J.S.	5.9	16.6	4.2	8.11	4.82	40.6	0.56	0.0093	4.35	3.92	9.9
30-W.B.	8.3	5.9	5.4	9.27	5.48	40.9	0.46	0.0133	2.73	2.48	9.3
31-J.K.	7.2	5.6	1.5	11.21	5.70	49.2	0.77	0.0077	3.51	2.66	24.2
32-E.G.	7.1	7.6	2.0	9.87	5.67	42.6	0.59	0.0103	2.51	1.97	21.4
Group mean	7.0	10.0	2.9	9.23	5.29	42.2	0.57	0.0105	3.17	2.68	15.8
±SE	±0.41	±2.26	±0.80	±0.633	±0.202	±1.94	±0.058	±0.00097	±0.339	±0.330	±3.02
F	1.29	0.25	0.27	0.64	1.06	1.04	0.11	0.20	0.66	0.54	1.51
Mean for all patients	6.6	10.3	2.6	8.99	5.38	40.0	0.55	0.0108	3.14	2.69	14.2
±SE	±0.13	±0.59	±0.22	±0.116	±0.070	±0.72	±0.015	±0.00037	±0.088	±0.082	±0.74
Normal mean	7.5	9.5	4.0	9.58	5.70	40.6	0.56	0.0111	3.39	2.88	15.1
±SE	±0.15	±0.53	±0.45	±0.076	±0.072	±0.35	±0.012	±0.00038	±0.105	±0.090	±0.76
P	<0.01	NS	<0.01	<0.001	<0.01	<0.01	<0.05	NS	NS	NS	NS

Although the percentage of plasma calcium bound to plasma protein was slightly above the upper limit of the normal range in five patients and slightly below the inferior limit in six, and hence the variability of protein-bound calcium in the investigated group was significantly greater than in the normal group ($p < 0.01$), the mean percentage, 40.0 ± 0.72, was almost the same as the normal mean 40.6 ± 0.35. The amount of calcium bound with one gram plasma protein was above the upper limit of the normal range in four of the 5 patients with a raised percentage of protein-bound calcium, and below the inferior limit in only one of the 6 patients with a lowered percentage of protein-bound calcium. Hence, the variability of this parameter in the group of investigated patients was significantly greater than that in the normal group ($p < 0.05$), although the means were almost the same: 0.55 ± 0.015 mg Ca/g protein and 0.56 ± 0.012 mg Ca/g protein, respectively. The dissociation constant K_{CaProt} was above the upper limit of the normal range in two patients only, and below the inferior limit in one patient only. The mean value and its variance of the investigated group, 0.0108 ± 0.00037 M, was almost the same as that of the normal group, 0.0111 ± 0.00038 M, which militates against an abnormal affinity of plasma proteins for binding calcium.

The plasma concentration of total inorganic phosphorus, 3.14 ± 0.088 mg/100 ml, was not significantly different from the normal mean, 3.39 ± 0.105 mg/100 ml, and all individual values were within the normal range. The plasma concentration of diffusible inorganic phosphorus, 2.69 ± 0.082 mg/100 ml, was not significantly different from the normal mean 2.88 ± 0.090 mg/100 ml, and only two patients had concentrations slightly above the upper limit of the normal range. Protein-binding of inorganic phosphate was 14.2 ± 0.74 per cent, which is almost the same as the normal mean 15.1 ± 0.76 per cent. Two patients had values above the upper limit and one below the lower limit of the normal range.

Renal Handling of Calcium and Inorganic Phosphate

Observed data in the patients have been given in Table 3 and Figs. 29—32. Since the analysis of variance of each parameter had not shown any significant difference between the subgroup means, the group has been treated as a single sample.

The mean glomerular filtration rate of water was 105.4 ± 5.52 ml/min. Only in three patients was the glomerular filtration rate below 75 ml/min, which is the inferior limit of the normal range, but in none was it below 40 ml/min, which is the limit beyond which renal failure influences renal ability to preserve phosphate (FRIIS et al., 1968).

In the first group of patients calcium clearance was normal in all but one (case 32-E.G.) with dysgerminoma of the ovary, in whom it was raised. The mean value for all patients was 2.2 ± 0.24 ml/min. The tubular reabsorption of calcium was normal in all but the above patient, in whom it was reduced. The mean value for all patients was 97.8 ± 0.19 per cent of the filtered load, and paralleled the level of diffusible calcium in plasma ultrafiltrate, according to the regression $y = 0.968\,x + 0.05$ ($r = 0.989$, $p < 0.001$), where y is the tubular reabsorption of calcium in mg per 100 ml filtrate, and x is the concentration of diffusible calcium in plasma ultrafiltrate in mg per 100 ml (Fig. 29). The non-reabsorbed part of the filtered calcium, that is, calcium excreted in urine, equalled 169 ± 14.7 mg/day. It was raised only in the patient with dysgerminoma of the ovary. The daily urinary calcium strictly paral-

Table 3. *Renal handling of calcium and inorganic phosphate*

Patient	GFR	C_{Ca}	U_{Ca}	T_{Ca}	C_{Pi}	U_{Pi}	T_{Pi}
	ml/min	ml/min	mg/day	%	ml/min	mg/day	%
1-M.B.	99.3	0.9	72	99.1	13.0	623	86.9
2-W.M.	120.1	2.3	185	98.1	11.2	421	90.6
3-M.L.	116.7	0.9	68	99.3	14.1	610	87.9
Group mean	112.0	1.4	108	98.8	12.8	551	88.5
±SE	±6.44	±0.47	±38.3	±0.37	±0.85	±65.3	±1.11
4-Z.S.	100.6	2.6	211	97.5	19.1	751	81.0
5-M.K.	62.8	3.0	189	95.2	17.2	836	72.7
6-K.A.	76.3	2.8	246	96.3	19.7	754	74.2
7-A.S.	146.6	4.5	296	96.9	10.2	672	93.0
8-E.J.	112.8	1.0	76	99.2	9.3	450	91.7
9-J.K.	173.6	1.8	136	98.9	17.7	918	89.8
10-J.C.	89.7	1.6	118	98.2	14.1	768	84.3
11-H.G.	91.9	2.5	201	97.3	11.4	540	87.6
12-M.N.	69.5	2.0	145	97.1	13.8	457	80.1
13-I.S.	81.6	1.4	120	98.2	9.3	535	88.6
14-B.G.	82.2	1.2	94	98.5	9.6	413	88.4
Group mean	98.9	2.2	167	97.6	13.8	645	84.7
±SE	±10.20	±0.30	±20.5	±0.36	±1.23	±52.1	±2.07
15-W.K.	72.4	1.5	107	97.9	8.5	442	88.2
16-B.K.	80.4	2.6	196	96.8	17.5	780	78.3
17-D.K.	121.9	1.9	145	98.5	14.6	620	88.0
18-S.W.	160.0	2.3	168	98.6	11.6	500	92.8
19-Z.G.	43.2	1.2	78	97.2	8.9	374	79.5
20-H.P.	129.2	1.8	143	98.6	21.2	745	83.6
21-W.O.	161.1	2.9	216	98.2	19.1	871	88.1
22-T.S.	138.9	3.3	271	97.6	21.6	932	84.5
23-H.B.	140.4	2.9	223	97.9	20.7	900	85.3
Group mean	116.4	2.3	172	97.9	16.0	685	85.4
±SE	±13.83	±0.24	±20.3	±0.21	±1.75	±69.6	±1.52
24-E.D.	81.1	0.9	71	98.9	9.6	485	88.1
25-M.G.	82.1	2.7	215	96.7	13.5	539	83.5
26-Z.S.	120.9	3.0	270	97.5	21.6	849	82.1
27-S.D.	122.7	2.1	171	98.3	17.4	734	85.8
Group mean	101.7	2.2	182	97.9	15.5	652	84.9
±SE	±11.61	±0.46	±42.1	±0.48	±2.58	±84.8	±1.32
28-K.C.	90.8	1.4	100	98.4	14.7	587	83.8
29-J.S.	75.0	0.8	52	99.0	8.2	533	89.1
30-W.B.	108.5	3.1	243	97.2	12.1	510	88.9
31-J.K.	120.3	1.9	153	98.4	11.3	509	90.6
32-E.G.	99.5	5.3	436	94.6	18.4	611	81.6
Group mean	98.8	2.5	197	97.5	12.9	550	86.8
±SE	±7.71	±0.80	±67.7	±0.79	±1.71	±20.8	±1.73
F	0.47	0.56	0.52	0.87	0.64	0.72	0.41
Mean for all patients	105.4	2.2	169	97.8	14.4	633	85.6
±SE	±5.52	±0.24	±14.7	±0.19	±0.76	±29.3	±0.88

GFR = true glomerular filtration rate; C_{Ca} and C_{Pi} = clearance, T_{Ca} and T_{Pi} = renal tubular reabsorption, and U_{Ca} and U_{Pi} = urinary excretion of calcium and phosphate, respectively; F = ratio of the between-subgroups variance estimate to the within-subgroups variance estimate.

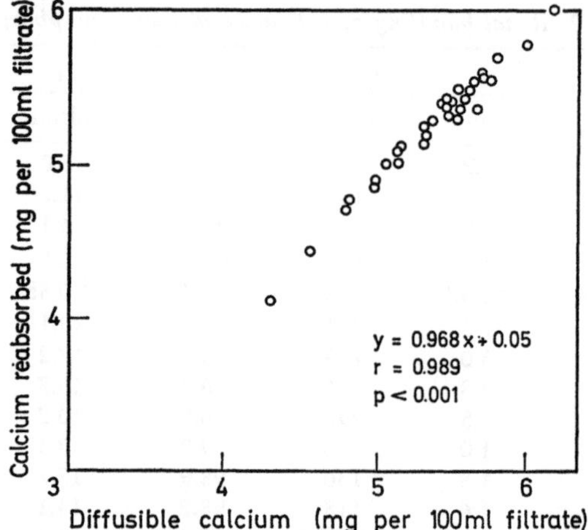

Fig. 29. The relation between tubular reabsorption of calcium per 100 ml filtrate and the concentration of diffusible calcium per 100 ml ultrafiltrate

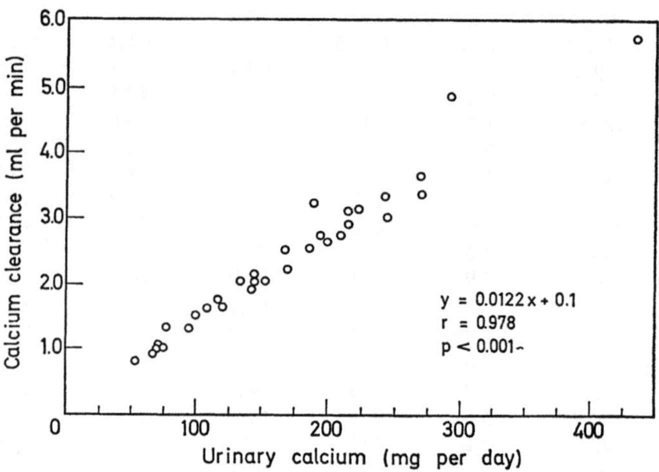

Fig. 30. The relation between calcium clearance and daily urinary calcium

leled the clearance of calcium, according to the regression $y = 0.122 x + 0.1$ ($r = 0.978$, $p < 0.001$), where y is the calcium clearance in ml/min, and x is the urinary calcium in mg/day (Fig. 30).

Of 32 patients, phosphate clearance was normal in 25 and raised in 7 patients. The mean value for all patients was 14.4 ± 0.76 ml/min. The tubular reabsorption of phosphate was normal in all but two patients. The mean value for all patients was 85.6 ± 0.88 per cent of the filtered load, and paralleled the level of diffusible phosphate in plasma ultrafiltrate, according to the regression $y = 0.997 x - 0.43$ ($r = 0.968$, $p < 0.001$), where y is the tubular reabsorption of phosphorus in mg per 100 ml filtrate, and x is the concentration of diffusible phosphorus in plasma ultrafiltrate in mg per 100 ml (Fig. 31). The non-reabsorbed part of the filtered phosphate, that is, phosphorus excreted in urine, was equal to 633 ± 29.3 mg/day. The urinary phos-

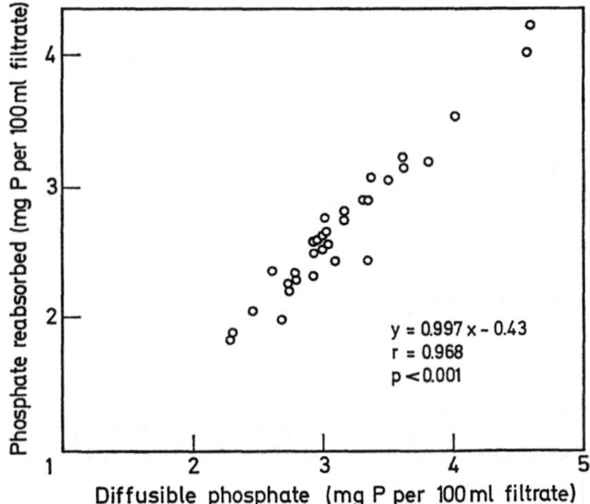

Fig. 31. The relation between tubular reabsorption of phosphate per 100 ml filtrate and the concentration of diffusible phosphate per 100 ml ultrafiltrate

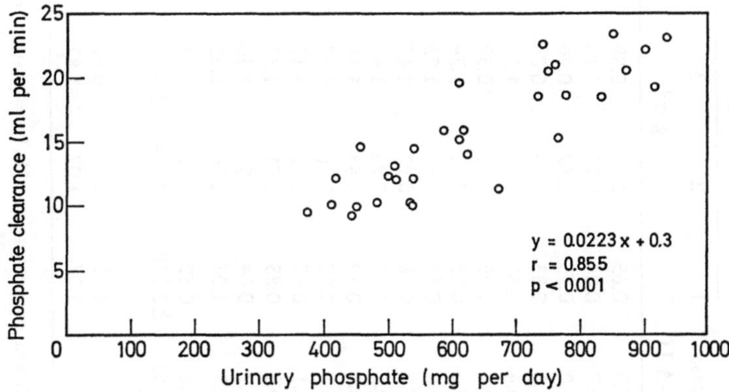

Fig. 32. The relation between phosphate clearance and daily urinary phosphate

phorus strictly paralleled the clearance of phosphorus, according to the regression $y = 0.0223 x + 0.3$ ($r = 0.855$, $p < 0.001$), where y is the phosphate clearance in ml/min, and x is the urinary phosphate in mg/day (Fig. 32).

Calcium Kinetics

The plasma data and the results of the compartmental analysis of calcium kinetics in 16 patients (second group) have been summarized in Table 4.

The mean plasma concentration of total calcium was 9.68 ± 0.132 mg/100 ml, that is, almost the same as the normal mean 9.58 ± 0.076 mg/100 ml. The mean plasma concentration of total inorganic phosphate was 3.19 ± 0.104 mg/100 ml, that is, almost the same as the normal mean 3.39 ± 0.105 mg/100 ml. The mean plasma concentration of alkaline phosphatase was 8.6 ± 0.51 King-Armstrong units/100 ml, that is, slightly lower than the normal mean 9.5 ± 0.53 K-A units/100 ml, though the difference is not significant.

Table 4. *Plasma values, compartment sizes, and flow constants of calcium*

Patient	BSA	[Ca]$_P$	[P$_i$]$_P$	Alk. P'tase	Compartment sizes				Flow constants			
					1	2	3	Total	ϱ_{01}	V_0^+	V_u	V_f
	m²	mg/100 ml		K-A U			g/m²			g/day·m²		
33-T.J.	1.41	9.80	3.60	7.5	0.65	0.87	0.89	2.41	0.460	0.287	0.099	0.074
34-T.J.	1.43	10.12	2.93	9.7	0.84	0.73	1.10	2.67	0.386	0.186	0.098	0.102
35-K.S.	1.42	8.78	3.16	8.0	0.75	0.67	0.76	2.18	0.524	0.351	0.105	0.068
36-P.M.	1.61	9.13	3.00	11.1	0.83	0.48	0.74	2.05	0.432	0.294	0.089	0.049
37-P.S.	1.43	9.30	3.02	6.4	0.67	0.70	1.36	2.73	0.504	0.309	0.075	0.120
38-B.J.	1.81	8.54	2.57	9.1	0.95	0.83	0.59	2.37	0.605	0.409	0.058	0.138
39-S.F.	1.87	10.27	4.28	7.6	0.85	0.53	1.74	3.12	0.513	0.316	0.083	0.114
40-W.J.	1.75	10.04	3.60	9.6	0.53	0.52	1.25	2.30	0.480	0.272	0.112	0.096
41-Z.A.	1.56	9.62	3.32	7.9	0.78	0.97	1.67	3.42	0.477	0.183	0.185	0.109
42-M.S.	1.75	9.90	2.67	9.5	1.07	0.90	1.41	3.38	0.713	0.412	0.198	0.103
43-W.H.	1.87	9.74	3.12	10.7	0.79	0.63	1.58	3.00	0.564	0.297	0.189	0.078
44-P.B.	1.80	10.25	3.18	6.5	0.92	0.36	1.87	3.15	0.507	0.372	0.037	0.098
45-O.S.	1.93	9.56	2.73	6.1	0.65	1.07	1.15	2.87	0.385	0.181	0.126	0.078
46-Z.W.	1.70	10.38	3.40	10.8	0.85	0.71	1.33	2.89	0.508	0.224	0.169	0.115
47-G.S.	1.73	9.64	3.18	5.2	0.64	0.91	1.20	2.75	0.388	0.167	0.129	0.092
48-G.W.	1.69	9.83	3.34	12.3	1.07	0.36	1.53	2.96	0.412	0.148	0.115	0.149
Mean	1.67	9.68	3.19	8.6	0.80	0.70	1.26	2.76	0.491	0.276	0.117	0.099
±SE	±0.044	±0.132	±0.104	±0.51	±0.038	±0.054	±0.094	±0.103	±0.0218	±0.0215	±0.0119	±0.0065
Range												
Lowest	1.41				0.53	0.36	0.59	2.05	0.385	0.148	0.037	0.049
Highest	1.93				1.07	1.07	1.87	3.42	0.713	0.412	0.198	0.149

BSA = body surface area; [Ca]$_P$ = plasma total calcium concentration; [P$_i$]$_P$ = plasma total inorganic phosphate concentration; ϱ_{01} = the rate of unidirectional calcium loss; V_0^+ = the calcium accretion rate; V_u = the urinary calcium excretion rate; V_f = the faecal endogenous calcium excretion rate.

Table 5. *Plasma values, compartment sizes, and flow constants of inorganic phosphate*

Patient	BSA	$[Ca]_P$	$[P_i]_P$	Alk. P'tase	Compartment sizes				Flow constants					
					1	2	3	Total	$\varrho_{12,21}$	$\varrho_{13,31}$	ϱ_{01}	ϱ_i	ϱ_u	ϱ_f
	m^2	mg/100 ml		K-A U		g/m^2						$g/day \cdot m^2$		
49-W.D.	1.84	8.96	4.04	8.6	0.45	1.04	7.62	9.11	2.74	2.92	1.498	0.901	0.509	0.088
50-K.D	1.69	9.02	4.48	12.4	0.67	1.31	7.20	9.18	5.37	3.49	1.419	0.979	0.367	0.073
51-P.J.	1.69	10.22	4.15	9.8	0.70	0.85	10.38	11.93	3.86	3.98	1.399	0.940	0.399	0.060
52-J.A.	1.79	9.77	3.16	9.5	0.78	1.75	9.37	11.90	5.32	3.79	1.522	0.934	0.508	0.080
53-J.M.	1.73	9.12	3.46	11.6	0.44	0.69	6.20	7.33	2.69	2.86	1.594	0.986	0.531	0.077
54-S.R.	1.68	9.30	3.82	7.3	0.51	1.20	5.43	7.14	4.08	2.89	1.513	1.074	0.369	0.070
55-A.M.	1.54	9.68	3.36	8.0	0.57	0.89	10.05	11.51	2.96	5.81	1.247	0.808	0.381	0.058
Mean	1.71	9.44	3.78	9.6	0.59	1.10	8.04	9.73	3.86	3.68	1.456	0.946	0.438	0.072
±SE	±0.036	±0.176	±0.180	±0.70	±0.050	±0.134	±0.730	±0.783	±0.433	±0.395	±0.0427	±0.0310	±0.0281	±0.0040
Range														
Lowest	1.54				0.44	0.69	5.43	7.14	2.69	2.86	1.247	0.808	0.367	0.058
Highest	1.84				0.78	1.75	10.38	11.93	5.37	5.81	1.594	1.074	0.531	0.088

BSA = body surface area; $[Ca]_P$ = plasma total calcium concentration; $[P_i]_P$ = plasma total inorganic phosphate concentration; $\varrho_{12,21}$, $\varrho_{13,31}$ = the rates of phosphate exchange between the respective compartments; ϱ_{01} = the rate of unidirectional phosphate loss; ϱ_i = the rate of internal loss of phosphate; ϱ_u = the urinary phosphate excretion rate; ϱ_f = the faecal endogenous phosphate excretion rate.

The mean size of the exchangeable calcium pool was 2.76 ± 0.103 g Ca/m^2 of body surface area, of which Compartment 1 comprised 0.80 ± 0.038 g/m^2, Compartment 2 0.70 ± 0.054 g/m^2, and Compartment 3 1.26 ± 0.094 g/m^2. The mean outflow of calcium from the exchangeable calcium pool was 0.491 ± 0.0218 g/m^2 per day, of which 0.276 ± 0.0215 g/m^2 per day represented bone accretion rate, and 0.117 ± 0.0119 g/m^2 per day urinary excretion, and 0.099 ± 0.0065 g/m^2 per day the faecal excretion of endogenous calcium.

Inorganic Phosphate Kinetics

The plasma data and the results of the compartmental analysis of inorganic phosphate kinetics in 7 patients (third group) have been summarized in Table 5.

The mean plasma concentration of total calcium was 9.44 ± 0.176 mg/100 ml, that is, almost the same as the normal mean 9.58 ± 0.076 mg/100 ml. The mean plasma concentration of total inorganic phosphate was 3.78 ± 0.180 mg/100 ml, that is, slightly higher than the normal mean 3.39 ± 0.105 mg/100 ml; the difference is not significant. The mean plasma concentration of alkaline phosphatase was 9.6 ± 0.70 King-Armstrong units/100 ml, that is, almost the same as the normal mean 9.5 ± 0.53 K-A units/100 ml.

The mean size of the exchangeable inorganic phosphate pool was 9.73 ± 0.783 g phosphorus/m^2 of body surface area, of which Compartment 1 comprised 0.59 ± 0.050 g/m^2, Compartment 2 1.10 ± 0.134 g/m^2, and Compartment 3 8.04 ± 0.730 g/m^2. The mean rate of phosphate exchange between Compartment 1 and Compartment 2 was 3.86 ± 0.433 g/m^2 per day, and almost the same was the mean rate of exchange between Compartment 1 and Compartment 3 (3.68 ± 0.395 g/m^2 per day). The outflow of phosphate from the exchangeable phosphate pool was 1.456 ± 0.0427 g/m^2 per day, of which 0.946 ± 0.0310 g/m^2 per day represented the internal loss, 0.438 ± 0.0281 g/m^2 per day—the urinary excretion, and 0.072 ± 0.0040 g/m^2 per day—the faecal excretion of endogenous phosphate.

2. Effects of Castration on Plasma State and Renal Handling of Calcium and Inorganic Phosphate

2.1. Clinical Material

The series consists of 17 patients, 14 fertile or pre-menopausal and 3 post-menopausal women, on whom bilateral X-ray castration was performed. Carcinoma of the uterine cervix was diagnosed in 15, and other cancers in 2 patients. The diagnoses are listed in Table 6.

2.2. Results

The plasma data before and after castration are shown in Table 7.

After castration, the concentration of plasma protein fell in 13 out of 17 patients, the mean going down from 6.5 ± 0.20 to 6.2 ± 0.18 g/100 ml. Although the mean difference ($d = -0.3 \pm 0.20$ g/100 ml) was not significant, the fact that protein concentration fell in 13 out of 17 patients is itself significant according to the sign test ($p < 0.05$, one-tail test). The effect of castration on plasma protein has been presented in Fig. 33.

The changes in plasma level of alkaline phosphatase were not consistent in either direction although, after castration, on the average they rose ($d = +1.8 \pm 1.42$ King-

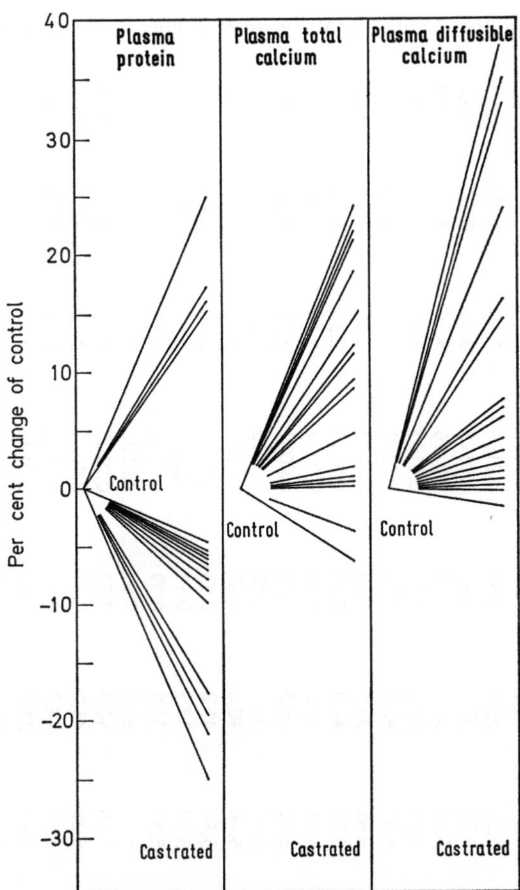

Fig. 33. Changes in plasma concentrations of protein (left), total calcium (middle), and diffusible calcium (right) following castration. Values are expressed in per cent change of control

Table 6. *Clinical data of patients subjected to castration*

Patient	Age (years)	Diagnosis
1-A.K.	56	Carcinoma of the uterine cervix, st. I
2-E.J.	35	Carcinoma of the uterine cervix, st. I
3-J.C.	47	Carcinoma of the uterine cervix, st. I
4-H.G.	27	Carcinoma of the uterine cervix, st. I
5-J.B.	50	Carcinoma of the uterine cervix, st. I
6-B.G.	37	Carcinoma of the uterine cervix, st. I
7-I.S.	43	Carcinoma of the uterine cervix, st. I
8-D.K.	37	Carcinoma of the uterine cervix, st. II
9-W.O.	34	Carcinoma of the uterine cervix, st. II
10-Z.G.	50	Carcinoma of the uterine cervix, st. II
11-W.K.	43	Carcinoma of the uterine cervix, st. II
12-A.K.	43	Carcinoma of the uterine cervix, st. II
13-M.G.	46	Carcinoma of the uterine cervix, st. III
14-Z.S.	44	Carcinoma of the uterine cervix, st. III
15-J.W.	46	Carcinoma of the uterine cervix, st. III
16-J.S.	20	Mesothelioma of the peritoneum
17-W.B.	27	Cancer of the ovary, after right oophorectomy

Table 7. *The effects of castration on the indices of bone dynamics and on the plasma state of calcium and inorganic phosphate*

Patient	Period of study	Plasma Protein	Alk. P'tase	Urinary PP_i	$[Ca]_P$	$[Ca]_D$	Ca_{PB}		K_{CaProt}	$[P_i]_P$	$[P_i]_D$	P_{PB}
		g/100 ml	K-A U	mg/day	mg/100 ml		%	mg/g protein	M	mg/100 ml		%
1-A.K.	A	6.3	34.7	0.4	8.25	4.03	51.2	0.67	0.0063	4.00	3.61	9.7
	B	6.0	19.4	0.7	8.59	5.32	38.1	0.55	0.0106	2.10	1.89	10.1
2-E.J.	A	6.8	7.2	2.4	8.87	5.55	37.4	0.49	0.0125	3.33	2.87	13.8
	B	5.6	6.3	3.4	8.94	5.87	34.3	0.55	0.0116	3.16	2.73	13.5
3-J.C.	A	7.2	7.0	1.9	9.07	5.16	43.1	0.54	0.0103	3.80	3.24	14.7
	B	6.6	15.8	0.8	10.97	6.29	42.7	0.71	0.0092	3.22	2.92	9.2
4-H.G.	A	6.4	6.4	2.1	9.32	5.61	39.8	0.58	0.0104	3.30	2.84	14.1
	B	7.3	11.6	2.5	9.35	5.53	40.9	0.53	0.0115	2.30	1.96	14.7
5-J.B.	A	6.3	8.0	1.6	8.68	5.05	41.8	0.58	0.0094	2.63	2.26	14.0
	B	7.2	11.9	2.0	10.48	5.40	48.5	0.71	0.0080	3.71	3.16	14.7
6-B.G.	A	5.6	9.5	1.3	8.38	5.47	34.7	0.52	0.0115	3.00	2.59	13.5
	B	5.3	7.5	1.4	9.10	5.46	40.0	0.69	0.0083	3.80	3.38	11.0
7-I.S.	A	7.9	8.8	3.0	9.97	5.80	41.8	0.53	0.0120	3.81	3.39	11.0
	B	6.0	18.2	2.6	9.39	5.87	37.5	0.59	0.0107	2.97	2.56	13.8
8-D.K.	A	7.1	10.9	2.2	8.13	5.38	33.8	0.39	0.0156	3.31	2.51	24.2
	B	6.7	8.7	8.7	9.52	5.59	41.3	0.59	0.0102	3.08	2.72	11.6
9-W.O.	A	6.7	8.3	6.1	8.64	5.16	40.3	0.52	0.0108	3.16	2.71	14.4
	B	6.4	11.1	2.9	9.58	5.27	45.0	0.67	0.0087	2.85	2.53	11.4
10-Z.G.	A	6.2	11.6	1.8	8.26	4.57	44.7	0.60	0.0082	2.93	2.52	14.0
	B	5.9	17.4	1.8	9.33	6.19	33.7	0.53	0.0126	3.32	2.86	13.7
11-W.K.	A	6.0	12.2	2.0	9.35	5.00	46.5	0.73	0.0072	3.60	3.10	13.8
	B	5.6	8.7	2.1	9.03	5.32	41.1	0.66	0.0085	2.00	1.73	13.5

PP_i = inorganic pyrophosphate; $[Ca]_P$ = plasma total calcium contentration; $[Ca]_D$ = plasma diffusible calcium concentration; Ca_{PB} = plasma protein-bound calcium; K_{CaProt} = dissociation constant of calcium proteinate; $[P_i]_P$ = plasma total inorganic phosphate concentration; $[P_i]_D$ = plasma diffusible inorganic phosphate concentration; P_{PB} = plasma protein--bound inorganic phosphate; A = control, B = after castration; $\overline{d} \pm S\overline{d}$ = mean and the standard error of mean of the changes from control; p = probability that mean of the changes is not different from zero, ascertained by one-tail t-test—values higher than 0.05 are non-significant (NS).

Table 7 (continued)

Patient	Period of study	Plasma Protein	Alk. P'tase	Urinary PP$_i$	[Ca]$_P$	[Ca]$_D$	Ca$_{PB}$		K$_{CaProt}$	[P$_i$]$_P$	[P$_i$]$_D$	P$_{PB}$
		g/100 ml	K-A U	mg/day	mg/100 ml		%	mg/g protein	M	mg/100 ml		%
12-A.K.	A	5.8	9.7	5.0	8.54	5.15	39.7	0.58	0.0095	3.20	2.94	8.2
	B	5.4	13.4	1.1	9.23	5.84	36.7	0.63	0.0099	4.10	3.64	11.2
13-M.G	A	5.5	8.9	3.1	9.06	5.55	38.8	0.64	0.0092	2.57	2.40	6.7
	B	6.7	10.3	6.0	9.10	5.71	37.3	0.51	0.0123	4.00	3.56	10.9
14-Z.S.	A	7.5	9.5	2.7	9.52	6.17	35.2	0.45	0.0153	2.73	2.32	14.9
	B	7.2	15.8	1.4	11.43	7.08	38.1	0.60	0.0125	2.73	2.33	14.7
15-J.W.	A	5.8	10.0	5.1	8.71	5.15	40.9	0.61	0.0090	2.40	1.99	17.2
	B	4.9	10.8	0.9	8.87	5.16	41.8	0.76	0.0070	3.10	2.70	13.0
16-J.S.	A	5.9	16.6	4.2	8.11	4.82	40.6	0.56	0.0093	4.35	3.92	9.9
	B	6.7	7.9	3.5	9.81	5.67	42.2	0.62	0.0098	3.95	3.47	12.2
17-W.B.	A	8.3	5.9	5.4	9.27	5.48	40.9	0.46	0.0133	2.73	2.48	9.3
	B	6.9	10.5	2.3	10.32	5.51	46.6	0.70	0.0083	2.02	1.57	22.5
Mean ± SE	A	6.5	10.3	3.0	8.83	5.24	40.7	0.56	0.0106	3.23	2.81	13.1
		±0.20	±1.58	±0.39	±0.130	±0.129	±1.11	±0.021	±0.00065	±0.133	±0.125	±0.97
	B	6.2	12.1	2.6	9.59	5.71	40.3	0.62	0.0100	3.08	2.69	13.0
		±0.18	±0.96	±0.49	±0.189	±0.114	±0.98	±0.018	±0.00042	±0.168	±0.155	±0.72
$\overline{d} \pm S\overline{d}$		−0.3	+1.8	−0.4	+0.76	+0.47	−0.4	+0.06	−0.0006	−0.15	−0.12	−0.1
		±0.20	±1.42	±0.62	±0.193	±0.134	±1.44	±0.028	±0.00072	±0.67	±0.209	±1.27
p		NS	NS	NS	<0.001	<0.001	NS	<0.05	NS	NS	NS	NS

Armstrong units per 100 ml), going up from 10.3 ± 1.58 to 12.1 ± 0.96 K-A units per 100 ml. The daily urinary pyrophosphate was also not consistent in either direction although, after castration, on the average it fell ($\bar{d} = -0.4 \pm 0.62$ mg per day), going down from 3.0 ± 0.3 to 2.6 ± 0.49 mg/day. The mean differences of each parameter were not significant. Instead, the changes in plasma concentration of alkaline phosphatase and daily urinary pyrophosphate were inversely related: a fall (or rise) in alkaline phosphatase level was accompanied by an increment (or reduction) in pyrophosphate excretion. This inversely related trend of changes due to castration was significant according to the sign test ($p < 0.05$, one-tail test).

After castration, the plasma concentration of total calcium rose in 15 out of 17 patients, crossing in three cases the upper limit of the normal range. The mean concentration rose from a control value of 8.83 ± 0.130 mg/100 ml to a value of 9.59 ± 0.189 mg/100 ml; the rise was highly significant ($\bar{d} = +0.76 \pm 0.193$ mg/100 ml; $p < 0.001$). The plasma concentration of diffusible calcium also rose in 14 out of 17 patients, crossing the upper limit of the normal range in three cases. This parameter fell in one case only, and did not change in two others. The mean concentration rose from a control value of 5.24 ± 0.129 mg/100 ml to a value of 5.71 ± 0.114 mg per 100 ml. The rise was highly significant ($\bar{d} = +0.47 \pm 0.134$ mg/100 ml; $p < 0.001$). It should be emphasized that the mean plasma concentrations of total and diffusible calcium after castration were almost the same as the normal means (cf. Table 2). The effect of castration on plasma concentration of total and diffusible calcium has been presented in Fig. 33.

The effect of castration upon protein-binding of calcium, expressed as percentage of calcium bound, gave random distribution of changes, and hence, the means were the same before as well as after castration ($\bar{d} = -0.4 \pm 1.44$ per cent; non-significant). A slight rise in amount of calcium bound by one gram of plasma protein ($\bar{d} = +0.06 \pm 0.028$ mg Ca/g protein; $p < 0.05$) was due to the rise in plasma level of calcium and the fall in plasma level of protein, since the calcium-binding ability of plasma protein expressed as K_{CaProt} did not change significantly ($\bar{d} = -0.0006 \pm 0.0072$ M).

The small changes in plasma concentration of total inorganic phosphate were not consistent in either direction although the mean fell after castration ($\bar{d} = -0.15 \pm 0.67$ mg/100 ml; non-significant). The changes in plasma concentration of diffusible phosphate paralleled those of total phosphate, and the mean also fell insignificantly ($\bar{d} = -0.12 \pm 0.209$ mg/100 ml). The effect of castration on protein-binding of phosphate, expressed as percentage of phosphate bound, gave random distribution of changes and, therefore, the means were the same before as well as after castration ($\bar{d} = -0.1 \pm 1.27$ per cent; non-significant).

The urinary data before and after castration are shown in Table 8, and Figures 34—37.

The changes in true glomerular filtration rate of water were not consistent in either direction although the mean rate fell after castration ($\bar{d} = -8.1 \pm 7.75$ ml/min; non-significant). Although in 10 out of 17 patients the renal clearance of calcium rose, the changes were so variable in quantity that the mean calcium clearance fell ($\bar{d} = -0.2 \pm 0.35$ ml per min; non-significant). The tubular reabsorption of filtered calcium did not change ($\bar{d} = -0.1 \pm 0.28$ per cent; non-significant) and paralleled the concentration of diffusible calcium in plasma ultrafiltrate, according to the regression $y = 1.003 \, x - 0.15$ ($r = 0.994$; $p < 0.001$), where y is the tubular reabsorption of

Table 8. *The effects of castration on renal handling of calcium and inorganic phosphate*

Patient	Period of study	GFR	C_{Ca}	U_{Ca}	T_{Ca}	C_{Pi}	U_{Pi}	T_{Pi}
		ml/min	ml/min	mg/day	%	ml/min	mg/day	%
1-A.K.	A	63.1	1.6	93	97.4	7.5	451	88.2
	B	61.4	1.6	121	97.4	11.7	368	81.0
2-E.J.	A	112.8	1.0	76	99.2	9.3	450	91.7
	B	85.9	1.3	112	98.5	9.0	408	89.6
3-J.C.	A	89.7	1.6	118	98.2	14.1	768	84.3
	B	72.9	2.1	193	97.1	11.0	541	84.9
4-H.G.	A	91.9	2.5	201	97.3	11.4	540	87.6
	B	90.7	2.8	223	96.9	21.4	708	76.4
5-J.B.	A	73.4	1.1	77	98.6	6.7	254	90.9
	B	61.6	2.2	169	96.5	11.1	593	82.0
6-B.G.	A	82.2	1.2	94	98.5	9.6	413	88.4
	B	87.3	1.7	131	98.1	6.0	339	93.1
7-I.S.	A	81.6	1.4	120	98.2	9.3	535	88.6
	B	83.0	1.3	108	98.5	18.6	797	77.6
8-D.K.	A	121.9	1.9	145	98.5	14.6	620	88.0
	B	111.1	2.1	169	98.1	13.3	610	88.0
9-W.O.	A	161.1	2.9	216	98.2	19.1	871	88.1
	B	96.7	3.7	283	96.1	15.1	638	84.4
10-Z.G.	A	43.2	1.2	78	97.2	8.9	374	79.5
	B	73.7	0.7	66	99.0	10.6	509	85.6
11-W.K.	A	72.4	1.5	107	97.9	8.5	442	88.2
	B	76.0	1.0	74	98.7	18.9	543	75.2
12-A.K.	A	133.5	4.2	314	96.8	14.9	728	88.9
	B	65.5	1.3	113	98.0	7.0	424	89.3
13-M.G.	A	82.1	2.1	215	96.7	13.5	539	83.5
	B	118.6	3.3	273	97.2	9.3	555	92.2
14-Z.S.	A	120.9	3.0	270	97.5	21.6	849	82.1
	B	92.0	1.3	138	98.5	15.1	593	83.6
15-J.W.	A	90.1	5.7	423	93.7	18.6	616	79.4
	B	42.1	1.9	142	95.5	6.7	300	84.1
16-J.S.	A	75.0	0.8	52	99.0	8.2	533	89.1
	B	103.0	2.2	178	97.9	10.7	627	89.6
17-W.B.	A	108.5	3.1	243	97.2	12.1	510	88.9
	B	143.1	4.0	317	97.2	26.4	697	81.5
Mean	A	94.3	2.2	167	97.7	12.2	558	86.8
$\pm$SE		$\pm$7.01	$\pm$0.31	$\pm$24.7	$\pm$0.31	$\pm$1.07	$\pm$40.7	$\pm$0.73
	B	86.2	2.0	165	97.6	13.1	544	84.6
		$\pm$5.88	$\pm$0.23	$\pm$17.6	$\pm$0.24	$\pm$1.36	$\pm$33.6	$\pm$1.29
$\bar{d}$		-8.1	-0.2	-2	-0.1	$+0.9$	-14	-2.2
$\pm$S$\bar{d}$		$\pm$7.75	$\pm$0.35	$\pm$26.1	$\pm$0.28	$\pm$1.76	$\pm$49.1	$\pm$1.60
p		NS	NS	NS	NS	NS	NS	NS

GFR = true glomerular filtration rate; C_{Ca} and C_{Pi} = clearance, T_{Ca} and T_{Pi} = renal tubular reabsorption, and U_{Ca} and U_{Pi} = urinary excretion of calcium and phosphate, respectively; A = control, B = after castration; $\bar{d}\pm$S$\bar{d}$ = mean and the standard error of mean of the changes from control; p = probability that the mean of the changes is not different from zero, ascertained by one-tail t-test, values higher than 0.05 are nonsignificant (NS).

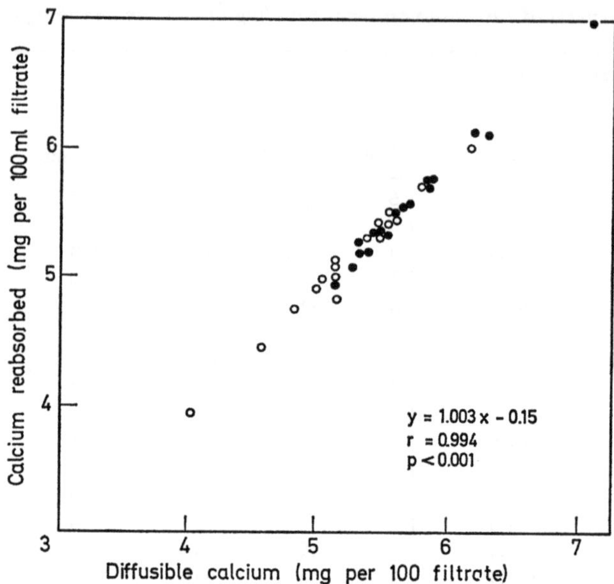

Fig. 34. The relation between tubular reabsorption of calcium per 100 ml filtrate and the concentration of diffusible calcium per 100 ml ultrafiltrate in patients before (○) and after (●) castration

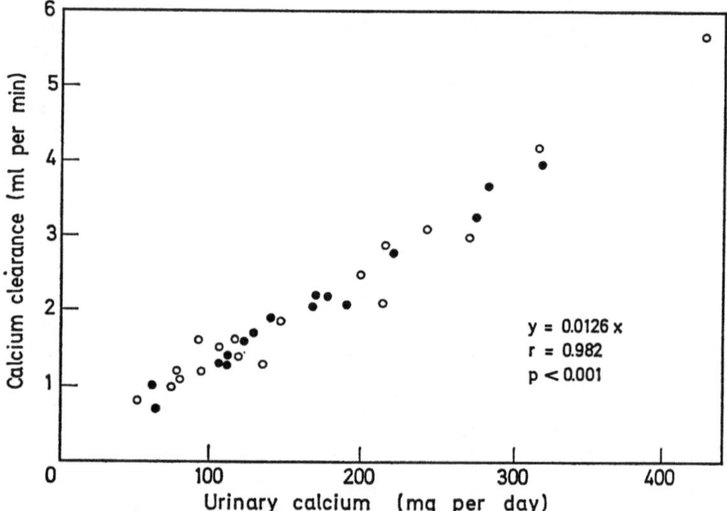

Fig. 35. The relation between calcium clearance and daily urinary calcium in patients before (○) and after (●) castration

calcium in mg per 100 ml filtrate, and x is the concentration of diffusible calcium in plasma ultrafiltrate in mg per 100 ml (Fig. 34). Since the reabsorbed calcium represented the same fraction of filtered calcium before and after castration, calcium clearance closely related to urinary calcium, according to the regression $y = 0.0126\,x$ ($r = 0.982$; $p < 0.001$), where y is calcium clearance in ml/min, and x is the excretion rate of calcium in urine in mg/day (Fig. 35).

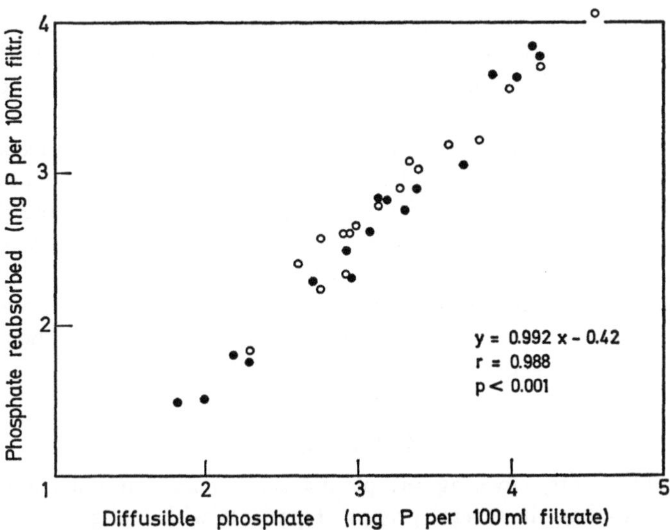

Fig. 36. The relation between tubular reabsorption of phosphate per 100 ml filtrate and the concentration of diffusible phosphate in ultrafiltrate in patients before (○) and after (●) castration

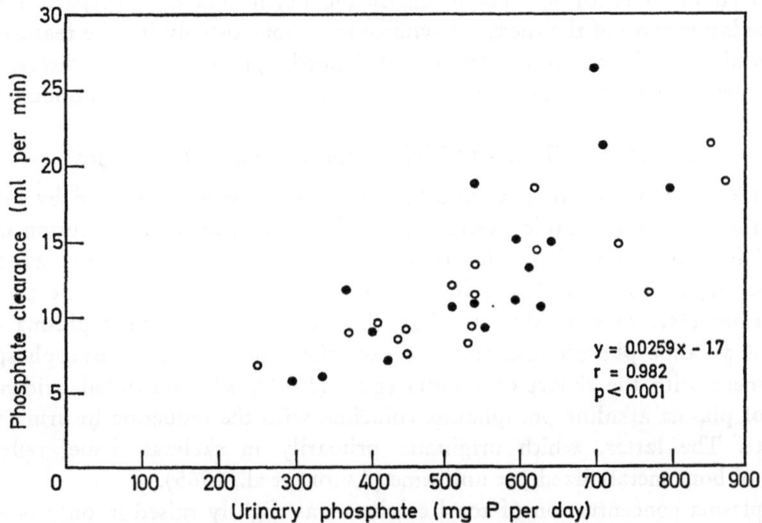

Fig. 37. The relation between phosphate clearance and daily urinary phosphate in patients before (○) and after (●) castration

The changes in renal handling of inorganic phosphate were as inconsistent as those of calcium, although somewhat greater than the latter. The changes in phosphate clearance were not consistent in either direction although the mean rose ($\bar{d} = +0.9 \pm$ 1.76 ml/min; non-significant). Tubular reabsorption of filtered phosphate rose in 4 and either did not change or fell in 13 out of 17 patients, the mean going down from 86.8 ± 0.73 to 84.6 ± 1.29 per cent of the filtered load ($\bar{d} = -2.2 \pm 1.60$ per cent; non-significant). But, this paralleled the concentration of diffusible phosphate in plasma ultrafiltrate, according to the regression $y = 0.992\,x - 0.42$ $(r = 0.988;\ p < 0.001)$, where y is the tubular reabsorption of phosphate in mg per 100 ml filtrate, and x is the concentration of diffusible phosphate in plasma ultrafiltrate in mg per 100 ml (Fig. 36).

Phosphate clearance was related to daily urinary phosphate, according to the regression $y = 0.0259\,x - 1.7$ $(r = 0.982;\ p < 0.001)$, where y is the phosphate clearance in ml/min, and x is the excretion rate of phosphate in urine in mg/day (Fig. 37). The scatter of values in this scattergram is greater than in the previous diagrams, since the fractional reabsorption of filtered phosphate represented somewhat different values for the control and post-castration periods. Of course, the changes in urinary excretion of phosphate were also inconsistent in either direction, although the mean fell insignificantly ($\bar{d} = -14 \pm 49.1$ mg per day).

3. Discussion

The present results, covering the plasma state, renal handling, and kinetics of calcium and phosphate in several groups of patients with malignancy without bone destruction, contribute some new findings upon bone mineral metabolism. It has not been the aim of this investigation to display the disturbances in bone mineral metabolism, resulting from elaboration by cancer of either the parathyroid hormone or osteolytic sterols. The former evolves the chemical syndrome of hyperparathyroidism, while the latter evolves the chemical syndrome of bone osteolysis. The features of the above syndromes do not differ from well-defined signs of common diseases, which have been the subject of widespread interest and a great number of publications.

3.1. Plasma State of Calcium and Inorganic Phosphate

The rather high level of plasma alkaline phosphatase accompanied by low daily excretion of urinary inorganic pyrophosphate indicates that bone resorption was well balanced by bone formation. This is not surprising, since all patients were in the fertile period, in which both the formation and the resorption of bone proceed at normal rates (MEEMA and MEEMA, 1968). The coincidence of high plasma concentration of alkaline phosphatase and low excretion rate of urinary pyrophosphate is in agreement with the report of AVIOLI et al. (1966), who presented evidence that the rise of plasma alkaline phosphatase coincides with the reduction in urinary pyrophosphate. The latter, which originates primarily in skeletal tissue, reflects the quantity of bone metabolized per unit time (AVIOLI et al., 1965).

The plasma concentration of total calcium was slightly raised in only one out of 3 patients with ovarian cancers considered as hormonally inactive. Ovarian cancers have been known to produce hypercalcaemia, although the number of patients so far known with this malignancy and hypercalcaemia was too small and the laboratory data too scanty to elucidate the mechanism of the mineral disturbances (PLIMPTON and GELLHORN, 1956; SEIFERT and SEEMANN, 1967). It should be stressed that plasma concentrations of diffusible calcium as well as total and diffusible phosphate were normal in each of 3 patients with ovarian cancer, and that the higher protein binding of calcium (and phosphate too) due to the higher calcium binding ability of plasma protein might be the reason for hypercalcaemia. PLIMPTON and GELLHORN (1956) suggested that ovarian cancer might produce an abnormal calcium binding substance and resemble the situation in laying hens. Recent work speaks for this concept. BENOWITZ and TEREPKA (1968) reported that most of calcium in hypercalcaemia induced in birds by oestradiol was complexed to de novo synthesized moiety of phosphoprotein, and PROCOPÉ (1969) showed that ovarian tumours generally considered as hormonally inactive were capable of producing higher-than-normal levels of oestrogens or their precursors. Obviously, further work is needed to elucidate the mechanism of hypercalcaemia in ovarian cancers considered as hormonally inactive.

In 13 of the remaining 29 patients the plasma concentration of total calcium was lowered and paralleled the also lowered concentration of diffusible calcium. Though the protein binding of calcium showed significantly higher variability in this group than in the normal one, the average value was almost the same in both groups. The dissociation constant of calcium proteinate indicated that the calcium binding ability of plasma protein was normal, and that the small disturbances in the protein binding of calcium were not due to any disturbance in the property of plasma protein, but due to simple variability in its concentration. The decrease in plasma concentration of calcium, both total and diffusible, is in agreement with the relatively high level of plasma alkaline phosphatase and with the relative reduction in urinary pyrophosphate. Recently, AVIOLI et al. (1966) observed a fall in pyrophosphate excretion accompanied by a decrease in plasma calcium and a rise in alkaline phosphatase during the postsurgical period in hyperparathyroidism, when bone destruction was presumably decreased while bone formation proceeded at rapid rate. The data obtained indicate that bone resorption in fertile women proceeds at relatively slow rate.

Raised plasma concentration of either total or diffusible plasma calcium has been reported in many papers, but decreased concentrations have rarely been observed and have not attracted any great interest, except hypoparathyroidism. Because of rising interest in medullary (C-cell) carcinoma accompanied by hypercalcitonism, hypocalcaemia will attract greater interest.

The plasma concentrations of total and diffusible inorganic phosphate were normal in all patients, although they showed a trend toward lower than normal values, while protein binding of phosphate was normal. Since the level of plasma phosphate reflects the pool of phosphate extraneous to bone, and since only 16 per cent of phosphate entering the pool of exchangeable phosphate comes from bone stores (see phosphate kinetics), the plasma concentration of inorganic phosphate cannot reflect the small changes in bone phosphate metabolism.

3.2. Renal Handling of Calcium and Inorganic Phosphate

The true glomerular filtration rate of water was below the inferior limit of the normal range, i. e., below 75 ml/min, in only 3 out of 32 patients, and in only one of these three patients was it near to 40 ml/min. This indicates that normal renal handling of calcium and phosphate should be expected in the patients studied, since FRIIS et al. (1968) reported that very slight renal failure, that is, with creatinine clearance above 40 ml/min, does not influence the tubular reabsorption of phosphate.

Renal clearance of calcium ranged from 0.8 to 4.5 ml/min and paralleled strictly the urinary excretion of calcium, which covered the normal range. Only in one patient, with dysgerminoma of the ovary, was calcium clearance increased, paralleling the also increased excretion of calcium in the urine. Tubular reabsorption of calcium ranged from 95.2 to 99.3 per cent, and only in the patient with ovarian dysgerminoma was it insignificantly lowered to 94.6 per cent. The values obtained for calcium clearance were greater than the values of 1.4—3.9 ml/min, whereas tubular reabsorption was within the range of values of 95—99 per cent, reported by LOKEN and GORDAN (1959). A different daily intake of calcium and phosphate, and different technique of ultrafiltration may be responsible for these small differences, as emphasized by TRANSBØL et al. (1968).

Renal clearance of phosphate ranged from 8.2 to 21.6 ml/min and paralleled the urinary excretion of phosphate, which covered the range from 374 to 932 mg/day. Taking the values of 6—17 ml/min (STROTT and NUGENT, 1968) as the normal range for phosphate clearance, it may be stated that at least a third of the 32 patients showed raised clearance. The tubular reabsorption of phosphate ranged from 78.3 to 93.0 per cent, and only in two patients was it lower than the value of 78 per cent, taken as the inferior limit of the normal range (NORDIN and FRASER, 1960). Hence, the present data indicate that the studied patients had slight disturbances in renal clearance and urinary excretion of phosphate, but they did not exhibit any significant disturbance in tubular reabsorption of this ion. Greater clearance and urinary excretion of phosphate might be due to the breakup and enhanced resorption of cancer tissue.

The indices of bone dynamics and the plasma state of calcium reflected bone metabolism better than the renal tests. From the latter, only the tubular reabsorption seems to be a test of high diagnostic value, while renal clearance and urinary excretion of phosphate cover too large a range, probably due to neoplasmatic breakup of soft tissue.

3.3. Effects of Castration on Bone Mineral Metabolism

A relationship between oestrogen deficiency and osteoporosis was postulated by ALBRIGHT et al. (1941), and documented by WALLACH and HENNEMAN (1959). Since Albright's concept had erroneously assumed osteoblastic failure as the consequence of oestrogen deficiency, this is compatible with the failure to find a consistently lower calcium accretion rate in osteoporosis or to produce changes in the osteoporotic skeleton through oestrogen treatment (NORDIN, 1960; BRONNER et al., 1963; DE SOMER et al., 1964; DYMLING 1964; LAFFERTY et al., 1964). JOWSEY and GERSHON-COHEN (1964) in a microradiographic study have shown that the increased porosity of osteoporotic bone is the result of enhanced bone resorption in the presence of normal levels of bone formation. MEEMA et al. (1965) postulated a thesis that the development of postmenopausal and senile osteoporosis would be due to increased bone resorption caused by a decrease or cessation of ovarian production of oestrogens which appear to counteract excessive bone resorption by some unknown mechanism. Although the decrease or cessation of ovarian production of oestrogens as the cause of exaggerated bone resorption is beyond doubt, the mechanism through which the action may be mediated has not been elucidated. Among mammals, oestrogens appear to stimulate bone formation only in mice where these hormones stimulate the processes which promote differentiation in the bones of preosteoblasts into osteoblasts, although they have no effect on the functional capacity of individual osteoblasts to synthesize and form collagen (SIMMONS, 1966). In man it is resorption that is inhibited (LAFFERTY et al., 1964; KATZ and KAPPAS, 1968). KATZ (1968) has found that oestrogens administered to man increase the disappearance rate of radioactivity from plasma after ^{14}C-proline injection, but not after ^{3}H-hydroxyproline. Since the former amino acid is incorporated into synthesized collagen, this result supports the view that oestrogens are directly anabolic with respect to protein synthesis in bone, too.

The data obtained in this study suggest that X-ray castration enhances bone resorption, confirming previous studies (YOUNG and NORDIN, 1967; SZYMENDERA and MADAJEWICZ, 1967). The raised plasma concentrations of total and diffusible calcium are a corollary to this exaggerated resorption. Hypercalciuria, which results from the increased filtered load of calcium because of raised plasma concentration of diffusible calcium (SZYMENDERA and MADAJEWICZ, 1967), has been observed in majority of castrated women, but it has not occurred in patients in whom the glomerular filtration rate had significantly diminished. These observations are in line with earlier ones (YOUNG and NORDIN, 1967; SZYMENDERA and MADAJEWICZ, 1967). Plasma and urinary phosphate did not show any definite rise, which is in agreement with our previous report (SZYMENDERA and MADAJEWICZ, 1967) but not with those of others (YOUNG and NORDIN, 1967; YOUNG et al., 1968), since phosphate is in equilibrium not only with the bone pool affected by enhanced resorption but also with the large pool of organic phosphate. It is of interest that the response of postmenopausal patients to castration has not differed from that of fertile women. This observation agrees with the data of PROCOPÉ (1969) who has shown that a significant ovarian oestrogen production most frequently occurs when less than 5 years have elapsed since the last menstruation, which was the case in the above patients.

Finally, this study has revealed that the combined curie and X-ray therapy of cancer of the uterine cervix may be a factor triggering the development of osteoporosis. An early onset of menopause might bring about vertebral deformities 15 to 20 years postmenopausally when, in terms of chronological age, these women would be in their fifties or early sixties (MEEMA and MEEMA, 1968). This effect is being overlooked by oncologists.

3.4. Calcium Kinetics

The mean plasma concentrations of total calcium and phosphate and alkaline phosphatase were normal. The value of calcium was almost the same as the normal mean, presumably due to the preponderance of males in this sample.

In the present compartmental model of calcium kinetics the particular compartments, M_1, M_2 and M_3, represented the values of 29%, 25% and 46% of the total exchangeable pool, respectively, and were close to the values 27%, 22% and 51%, respectively, reported by RAYNAUD and KELLERSHOHN (1966). Two thirds of the calcium pool in Compartment 1, which exhibits the biological half-life of about 1 hour, represents the extracellular fluid, and the remaining third belongs to the most rapidly exchanging bone calcium and partly to the intracellular calcium (SZYMENDERA et al., 1967 b). Compartment 2, with a biological half-life of 1.5 hour, consists of both the remaining part of the intracellular calcium and a fraction of slowly exchanging bone calcium (AVIOLI and HENNEMAN, 1964). Compartment 3, with a biological half-life of 0.75 day, represents primarily the slowly exchanging bone calcium (AVIOLI and HENNEMAN, 1964) and some of the cartilage calcium and dystrophic tissue calcium (HEANEY, 1964). The total exchangeable calcium pool represents a biological half-life of about 4 days.

The mean value of the total exchangeable calcium pool, 2.76 g/m², is essentially the same as the mean of the reference standard for calcium turnover data, 2.77 g/m², constructed by HEANEY et al. (1964) and computed by COHN et al. (1965) with the SAAM programme. The average urinary excretion rate, 0.117 g/m² per day, is about 41% higher than the value of 0.083 g/m² per day of the reference standard, and about 20% higher than the mean value of fertile women, but lower than the mean value preported by NEER et al. (1967). The inspection of the urinary data presented in Table 4 reveals that the males showed distinctly greater excretion rates than the females, which agrees well with the results of ROSE (1966), wo reported higher excretion rates in males than in females, both in health and disease. The preponderance of males in the sample explains the trend toward the higher mean. The same might be true for the mean excretion rate of faecal endogenous calcium, 0.099 g/m² per day, which is 34% higher than the reference-standard value of 0.074 g/m² per day. The difference between the accretion rate of this study, 0.276 g/m² per day, and that of the reference standard, 0.224 g/m² per day, might have also been due to the above cause, since the malignant lesions did not include hormone-secreting tumours and, besides, they were too small to influence the overall body metabolism in general, and total calcium metabolism in particular. COHN et al. (1965) found in apparently normal subjects values covering the same range as those presented in this work.

It follows from the above data that the values presented in this study are in agreement with those for normal subjects obtained by other workers.

3.5. Phosphate Kinetics

The mean plasma concentrations of total calcium and phosphate and alkaline phosphatase were normal.

About 85% of body phosphate of an adult man can be accounted for by the skeleton (WIDDOWSON and DICKERSON, 1964). If one takes a value of 12 grams phosphorus per kilogram body weight (WIDDOWSON and DICKERSON, 1964), then there should be about 790 grams phosphorus in a subject weighing 66 kg (the mean weight of the patients studied), and of that value about 670 grams are in the skeleton and 120 grams in the soft tissues. The calculated body exchangeable phosphorus represents about 17 grams, that is, 2.2% of the body phosphate pool.

In the present compartmental model of phosphate kinetics the particular compartments, M_1, M_2 and M_3, represented the values of 6%, 11% and 83% of total exchangeable pool, respectively. Each compartment symbolizes a totality of particles within the system that are operationally indistinguishable from each other, and may or may not correspond to any identifiable physiological space (AVIOLI and BERMAN, 1966). Compartment 1 represents the site into which the tracer was injected and from which blood samples were drawn, and thus includes the extracellular space. The phosphate pool of extracellular fluid should be 0.42 g or 0.25 g/m² (these calculations assumed the plasma concentration of phosphate = 3.8 mg per 100 ml, the extracellular fluid volume = 0.17 body weight, and body weight = 66 kg), that is, it explains only a half of the pool, since Compartment 1 has 0.59 g/m². The turnover rate of this pool is relatively fast, with a biological half-life of about 1 hour, or, almost the same as in the case of calcium. It might be presumed that the remaining phosphate in Compartment 1 could represent the most rapidly exchanging bone phosphate and intracellular phosphate, as it does in calcium kinetics. Compartment 2 is the pool of phosphate that represents the intermediate turnover rate, with a biological half-life of about 5 hours, that is, thrice that of calcium. Compartment 3 represents the slow turnover rate, with a biological half-life of about 1.5 day, which is twice that of calcium. Since the exchangeability of phosphate with bone mineral seems to be similar to that of calcium within the weight ratio Ca/P from 1.84 to 2.16, it is probable that only about $30^0/0$ of the phosphate pool of Compartment 2 and about $7^0/0$ of Compartment 3 represents bone phosphate, while the bulk of the phosphate pool represents the soft tissue phosphate. The total exchangeable phosphate pool represents a biological half-life of about 4.5 days, that is, almost the same as calcium.

The intercompartmental flow constants between Compartment 1 and either lateral compartment are almost the same. The mean outflow of phosphate from the exchangeable pool was 1.456 g/m² per day, divided into several excretion rates. The mean excretion rate into urine was 0.438 g/m² per day and into faeces 0.072 g/m² per day. The rate of internal loss was 0.946 g/m² per day.

The latter could be subdivided into two components, as will be clear from the following. The calcium apatites range in Ca/P weight ratio from the theoretical value of 2.16, equivalent to a molar ratio 10-Ca to 6-P, down to a low value of 1.84, equivalent to a molar ratio 8.5-Ca to 6-P (POSNER, 1960). Since the newly deposited mineral is deficient in calcium, the low value of 1.84 seems to be the better approximation of the ratio of both elements accreted into bone. If the mean calcium accretion rate is 0.276 g calcium per m² per day, it has to be accompanied by 0.150 g phosphorus per m² per day. Thus, only about $16^0/0$ of the internally deposited phosphate is accreted into the bone mineral, while as much as $84^0/0$ is incorporated into other sites, presumably into long-living organic compounds.

Since there is remarkably little information regarding the kinetics of phosphate metabolism in man, especially, there is a lack of a reference standard, no conclusions can be drawn from these results. Nevertheless, the data suggest that exchangeable phosphate occupies the extraskeletal tissues in the first place, and that the bulk of phosphate leaving that pool is either excreted or converted into organic compounds.

The Metabolism of Bone Mineral in Malignancy with Bone Lesions

The association of alterations in plasma state, renal handling, and kinetics of calcium and inorganic phosphate with malignant bone lesions is a well-established phenomenon. However, the pathogenesis of these alterations is not uniform.

When a neoplasma has resided in the skeleton and effected widespread destruction of bone tissue, there is a possibility that the products of osteolysis released into the blood stream will result in an elevation of plasma concentration and urinary excretion of calcium and inorganic phosphate (LASZLO et al., 1952; LAZOR and ROSENBERG, 1964; MYERS et al., 1966; MUIRHEAD, 1967; MYERS et al., 1968). The reverse phenomenon, a decrease of plasma concentration and urinary excretion of calcium and inorganic phosphate, is observed in osteoblastic metastases (RANDALL and LIRENMAN, 1964) and during recalcification of the oesteolytic metastases (MUIRHEAD, 1967; SZYMENDERA et al., 1967 a). The finding of osseous metastases does not exclude the likelihood that simultaneously a calcium-mobilizing substance produced by the tumour itself, either a parathyroid hormone-like peptide (TASHJIAN et al., 1964) or a vitamin D-like sterol (GORDAN et al., 1966; GORDAN, 1967), is responsible for the abnormal bone mineral metabolism.

The disturbances in plasma state and renal handling of calcium and inorganic phosphate associated with plasmacytoma seem to be attributable to simple bone destruction by neoplasma (LAZOR and ROSENBERG, 1964). Of course, the skeletal lesions need not be accompanied by changes in plasma state and urinary excretion of bone mineral. Simultaneous osteolysis, from direct infiltration of bone by metastases and from elaboration of osteolytic substances by the tumour, seems to take place in patients with cancer of the breast (HORTON and OLSON, 1964).

The metabolism of bone mineral in the two essentially different neoplastic states has been the object of investigation and the results are presented in this chapter.

1. Patients with Plasmacytoma

1.1. Clinical Material

The material comprises 20 patients with plasmacytoma: 8 females and 12 males. All the patients, with widespread osteolytic lesions of the ribs, spine, pelvis, and other bones, were treated with X-rays and/or alkylating agents. Of the 20 patients, the plasma state and renal handling of calcium and inorganic phosphate were studied in sixteen; these studies have been repeated in several patients during consecutive admissions. The kinetics of calcium metabolism has been studied in two other patients, and the kinetics of inorganic phosphate metabolism in the two remaining ones.

1.2. Results

Plasma State of Calcium and Inorganic Phosphate

Observed data in 16 patients are given in Table 9. The mean pyrophosphate excretion in 16 normal subjects (AVIOLI and HENNEMAN, 1966), and the mean values of the remaining parameters in 25 normal subjects (SMARSZ, in press) have been also included. The group of patients studied was divided into 3 subgroups: the first subgroup comprises 21 studies in 11 patients without any signs of renal failure, the second, 13 studies in 8 patients with mild renal failure (6 patients of this subgroup belong also to the former one), and the third, 3 studies in 3 patients with moderate renal failure. Since the analysis of variance of each parameter had not shown any significant difference among the subgroup means, the group has been treated as a single sample.

Among the 16 patients, the concentration of plasma protein was below the inferior limit of the normal range in four, and above the upper limit of the normal range in four others. Although the mean concentration of plasma protein, 7.3 ± 0.23 g/100 ml (mean and SE), was almost the same as the normal mean, 7.5 ± 0.15 g/100 ml, the variance was significantly greater than that of the normal subjects ($p < 0.01$). It should be stressed that neither the decrease nor the rise of plasma protein concentration was a stable phenomenon: both were found four times in the 37 studies on 16 patients.

The plasma level of alkaline phosphatase exceeded the upper limit of the normal range in 5 patients, but only in two of them was it found to be raised during subsequent admissions. The mean concentration of alkaline phosphatase, 13.0 ± 0.74 King-Armstrong units/100 ml, was higher than the normal mean, 9.5 ± 0.53 K-A units/100 ml, and the variance was significantly greater than that of normal subjects ($p < 0.01$). The excretion of urinary inorganic pyrophosphate was slightly raised in two patients and normal in the remainder. The mean excretion, 3.0 ± 0.34 mg/day, was slightly lower than the normal mean, 4.0 ± 0.45 mg/day, but the variability of the studied group was significantly greater than that of the normal subjects ($p < 0.05$).

The plasma concentration of total calcium, 9.40 ± 0.146 mg/100 ml, was slightly lower than the normal mean, 9.58 ± 0.076 mg/100 ml, and the variance of total calcium concentration for this group was greater than that for the normal subjects ($p < 0.01$). In three patients the concentration was below the inferior limit of the normal range, and in two patients it exceeded the upper limit. It should be emphasized that the raised concentration of total calcium turned out to be lower during subsequent admissions (case 8-B.P.). The plasma concentration of diffusible calcium, 5.69 ± 0.075 mg/100 ml, was almost the same as the normal mean, 5.70 ± 0.072 mg per 100 ml. It exceeded the upper limit of the normal range in 5 studies of 4 patients, and fell below the inferior limit of the normal range in 4 patients; the plasma concentration of diffusible calcium in patient 8-B.P. has been found raised twice and lowered once. Nevertheless, the variance of concentrations in whole group did not differ from that of normal subjects.

The percentage of plasma calcium bound to plasma protein was above the upper limit of the normal range in two patients only, and below the inferior limit of the normal range in 7 patients. In two patients (cases 6-A.G. and 8-B.P.) the raised

Table 9. *Indices of bone dynamics and plasma state of calcium and inorganic phosphate in patients with plasmacytoma*

Patient and study		Sex and age	Plasma Protein	Alk. P'tase	Urinary PP_i	$[Ca]_P$	$[Ca]_D$	Ca_{PB}		K_{CaProt}	$[P_i]_P$	$[P_i]_D$	P_{PB}
		yrs	g/100 ml	K-A U	mg/day	mg/100 ml		%	mg/g protein	M	mg/100 ml		%
Patients without renal failure — GFR $>$ 75 ml/min													
1-S.K.	1	F 47	7.5	10.2	6.6	9.30	5.51	40.8	0.51	0.0119	4.80	4.08	14.9
2-S.K.	1	M 36	10.2	8.6	2.2	9.07	5.23	42.3	0.38	0.0156	2.84	2.53	10.8
3-K.K.	1	M 36	5.6	14.8	2.7	8.97	5.74	36.0	0.58	0.0107	2.66	2.57	3.5
	2		6.9	13.2	2.9	8.97	5.63	37.2	0.48	0.0074	2.90	2.48	14.5
4-F.S.	1	M 62	7.7	27.9	1.7	9.55	5.54	42.0	0.52	0.0128	4.15	3.69	11.1
	2		5.7	23.2	2.1	9.40	5.54	41.1	0.68	0.0059	3.70	3.28	11.4
5-T.S.	1	M 64	6.3	9.5	2.6	9.68	5.53	42.9	0.66	0.0089	2.47	2.18	11.6
	2		6.6	14.3	2.4	8.98	5.62	37.7	0.51	0.0121	2.17	1.95	10.1
	3		7.2	15.7	2.6	9.33	5.99	35.8	0.46	0.0143	2.20	2.01	8.6
6-A.G.	1	M 63	7.5	7.9	3.7	9.42	5.22	44.6	0.56	0.0101	3.20	3.02	5.6
7-A.K.	1	F 36	5.1	9.6	7.8	9.29	5.90	36.5	0.66	0.0094	4.44	3.43	22.7

PP_i = inorganic pyrophosphate; $[Ca]_P$ = plasma concentration of total calcium; $[Ca]_D$ = plasma concentration of diffusible calcium; Ca_{PB} = protein-bound plasma calcium; K_{CaProt} = dissociation constant of calcium proteinate; $[P_i]_P$ = plasma concentration of total inorganic phosphate; $[P_i]_D$ = plasma concentration of diffusible inorganic phosphate; P_{PB} = plasma protein-bound inorganic phosphate; F = ratio of the between-subgroups variance estimate to the within-subgroups variance estimate; p = probability that the means or variances for all patients and normal subjects are not different—values higher than 0.05 are nonsignificant (NS).

Table 9 (continued)

Patient and study		Sex and age	Plasma Protein	Alk. P'tase	Urinary PP_i	$[Ca]_P$	$[Ca]_D$	Ca_{PB}		K_{CaProt}	$[P_i]_P$	$[P_i]_D$	P_{PB}
		yrs	g/100 ml	K-A U	mg/day	mg/100 ml		%	mg/g protein	M	mg/100 ml		%
8-B.P.	1	M 58	6.7	12.8	2.0	13.06	6.48	50.4	0.98	0.0064	3.07	2.57	16.3
	2		4.9	7.0	2.0	8.52	4.89	42.6	0.74	0.0068	3.31	2.88	13.0
9-H.W.	2	F 53	7.8	13.3	4.1	9.20	5.50	40.2	0.47	0.0128	3.20	2.72	8.5
	3		7.5	16.6	1.6	9.32	5.92	36.5	0.45	0.0145	2.97	2.57	13.5
10-W.G.	2	F 50	8.0	12.4	1.4	9.71	5.47	43.7	0.53	0.0112	3.34	2.99	10.5
	3		8.5	14.7	2.0	9.42	5.90	37.4	0.41	0.0159	3.10	2.62	15.5
	4		9.4	14.0	1.6	8.85	5.54	37.4	0.35	0.0178	3.36	2.94	12.5
11-M.B.	3	F 57	6.6	6.6	4.0	9.23	6.03	34.7	0.48	0.0179	3.85	3.39	11.9
	4		7.4	19.8	10.3	8.94	5.79	35.2	0.43	0.0152	3.70	3.32	10.3
	5		7.6	20.2	2.6	9.10	5.22	42.6	0.51	0.0112	3.32	2.90	12.7
Group mean ±SE			7.2 ±0.28	13.9 ±1.18	3.3 ±0.50	9.39 ±0.194	5.63 ±0.076	39.9 ±0.86	0.54 ±0.031	0.0119 ±0.00079	3.27 ±0.127	2.86 ±0.118	11.9 ±0.86
Patients with mild renal failure — GFR 40—75 ml/min													
6-A.G.	2		8.5	10.8	1.6	9.97	6.37	36.1	0.42	0.0168	3.36	2.92	13.1
	3		8.5	11.7	1.9	9.42	5.88	37.6	0.42	0.0158	3.00	2.70	10.0
7-A.K.	2		6.0	16.6	5.2	9.16	5.63	38.5	0.59	0.0103	4.64	4.12	11.3
8-B.P.	3		6.7	13.3	1.8	9.39	6.14	34.6	0.49	0.0139	2.96	2.62	11.5
	4		6.3	13.3	1.8	9.10	5.64	38.0	0.55	0.0111	3.00	2.75	8.3
9-H.W.	1		6.9	16.8	2.9	9.77	5.82	40.4	0.57	0.0110	3.10	2.78	10.3
10-W.G.	1		6.7	9.8	7.9	7.63	4.46	41.5	0.47	0.0104	3.81	3.26	14.4

Table 9 (continued)

Patient and study		Sex and age	Plasma Protein	Alk. P'tase	Urinary PP_i	$[Ca]_P$	$[Ca]_D$	Ca_{PB}		K_{CaProt}	$[P_i]_P$	$[P_i]_D$	P_{PB}
		yrs	g/100 ml	K-A U	mg/day	mg/100 ml		%	mg/g protein	M	mg/100 ml		%
11-M.B.	1		6.8	15.2	0.9	9.11	5.61	38.4	0.51	0.0119	4.29	3.67	14.4
	2		6.2	11.6	1.7	8.60	5.38	37.4	0.52	0.0113	3.20	2.75	14.1
12-B.L.	1	M 45	7.7	11.8	2.5	10.22	5.89	42.4	0.56	0.0113	1.67	1.67	0
13-A.S.	1	F 61	8.8	9.8	1.3	9.44	5.79	38.5	0.41	0.0157	4.44	3.58	19.4
	2		7.1	11.3	2.6	8.91	5.59	37.3	0.47	0.0132	3.65	3.29	9.9
	3		9.0	11.7	3.0	9.62	5.94	38.2	0.41	0.0162	3.56	3.15	11.5
Group mean			7.3	12.6	2.7	9.26	5.70	38.4	0.49	0.0130	3.44	3.01	11.4
±SE			±0.29	±0.65	±0.52	±0.180	±0.125	±0.58	±0.018	±0.00066	±0.213	±0.177	±1.23
Patients with moderate renal failure — GFR 20—40 ml/min													
14-Z.U.	1	M 34	7.3	9.0	3.9	9.25	5.57	39.8	0.50	0.0121	4.19	3.66	12.8
15-J.W.	1	M 67	11.6	6.6	2.2	12.04	7.23	40.0	0.41	0.0195	3.32	2.66	19.9
16-J.W.	1	F 46	5.9	10.8	0.9	8.87	5.16	41.8	0.63	0.0087	3.10	2.67	13.9
Group mean			8.3	8.8	2.3	10.05	5.99	40.5	0.51	0.0134	3.54	3.00	15.5
±SE			±1.71	±1.22	±0.87	±1.000	±0.633	±0.64	±0.064	±0.00319	±0.333	±0.332	±2.21
F			0.82	1.86	0.47	0.98	0.73	1.04	0.69	0.62	0.38	0.29	1.27
Mean for all patients			7.3	13.0	3.0	9.40	5.69	39.4	0.52	0.0124	3.35	2.93	12.0
±SE			±0.23	±0.74	±0.34	±0.146	±0.075	±0.54	±0.019	±0.00055	±0.106	±0.093	±0.68
Normal mean			7.5	9.5	4.0	9.58	5.70	40.6	0.56	0.0111	3.39	2.88	15.1
±SE			±0.15	±0.53	±0.45	±0.076	±0.072	±0.35	±0.012	±0.00038	±0.105	±0.090	±0.76
P			<0.01	<0.01	<0.05	<0.01	NS	<0.01	<0.01	<0.01	NS	NS	<0.01

percentage of protein bound calcium turned out to be lower in subsequent studies. The variance of this parameter was significantly greater in the studied group than in the normal subjects ($p < 0.01$), although the means were almost the same and equal to 39.4 ± 0.54 per cent and 40.6 ± 0.35 per cent, respectively. The amount of calcium bound with one gram of plasma protein was above the upper limit of the normal range in one patient only; this raised value turned out to be lower on subsequent admission. The values of this parameter were below the inferior limit of the normal range in 8 studies of 5 patients; in 3 patients lower values were repeatedly found in consecutive admissions. Like the percentage of calcium bound to protein, the variance of this parameter was significantly greater in patients with plasmacytoma than in normal subjects ($p < 0.01$), although the means were almost the same and equal to 0.52 ± 0.019 and 0.56 ± 0.012 mg Ca/g protein, respectively. The dissociation constant K_{CaProt} was below the inferior limit of the normal range in two patients only (in 3 studies), and above the upper limit of the normal range in 6 others (in 4 patients the raised value was found twice). Hence, the mean and variance of K_{CaProt} were significantly greater than those of the normal subjects ($p < 0.01$). It militates in favour of an abnormal affinity of plasma protein for binding calcium, at least in some out of the patients with plasmacytoma.

The plasma concentration of total inorganic phosphate, 3.35 ± 0.106 mg/100 ml, was not significantly different from the normal mean, 3.39 ± 0.105 mg/100 ml. In two patients the concentration of total inorganic phosphate was above the upper limit of the normal range, and in two others (in 3 studies) it was below the inferior limit. The raised concentration of total phosphate was accompanied by a raised level of diffusible phosphate. On the other hand, the lowered concentration of total inorganic phosphate was accompanied by a lowered concentration of diffusible phosphate in only one patient whose protein binding of inorganic phosphate was practically equal to zero (case 12-B.L.). Hence, the plasma concentration of diffusible inorganic phosphate, 2.93 ± 0.093 mg/100 ml, was not significantly different from the normal mean, 2.88 ± 0.090 mg/100 ml. In 3 patients the protein-binding of inorganic phosphate was below the inferior limit of the normal range, and in the remainder it tended towards lower values. Therefore, the mean protein binding of inorganic phosphate, 12.0 ± 0.68 per cent, was significantly lower than the normal mean, 15.1 ± 0.76 per cent ($p < 0.01$).

The above data indicate that a very large range of values might be anticipated in the group of patients with plasmacytoma, although the bulk of the chemical data lies within the limits of the normal range.

Renal Handling of Calcium and Inorganic Phosphate

Observed data in 16 patients are given in Table 10 and Figs. 38—41. The group has been divided into subgroups according to the functional state of the kidneys, as mentioned. Therefore, the analysis of variance has shown the greatest difference among the subgroup means of the true glomerular filtration rate, and much smaller differences, or even the lack of any difference, among the subgroup means of renal tests of calcium and phosphate.

The mean value of the true glomerular filtration rate for all patients was 80.6 ± 4.69 ml/min, but it differed among the subgroups ($p < 0.001$). The mean value was 100.0 ± 3.86 ml/min in patients without renal failure, 62.1 ± 2.72 ml/min in

Table 10. *Renal handling of calcium and inorganic phosphate in patients with plasmacytoma*

Patient	Study	GFR ml/min	C_{Ca} ml/min	U_{Ca} mg/day	T_{Ca} %	C_{Pi} ml/min	U_{Pi} mg/day	T_{Pi} %
Patients without renal failure—GFR > 75 ml/min								
1-S.K	1	114.0	2.5	199	97.8	14.7	1016	87.1
2-S.K.	1	99.8	1.1	85	98.9	28.8	1264	71.1
3-K.K.	1	102.0	2.1	177	97.9	19.3	825	81.1
	2	101.2	1.1	93	98.9	17.1	714	83.1
4-F.S.	1	79.3	4.0	321	94.9	14.1	883	82.2
	2	125.0	10.0	794	92.0	19.5	1064	82.2
5-T.S.	1	105.1	2.5	196	97.7	24.4	890	76.8
	2	92.3	1.5	122	98.4	16.3	534	82.3
	3	144.2	2.2	191	98.5	24.0	815	83.4
6-A.G.	1	85.4	2.1	160	97.5	16.6	847	80.6
7-A.K.	1	121.7	1.1	92	99.1	16.3	928	86.6
8-B.P.	1	104.5	3.1	285	97.1	10.4	450	90.0
	2	74.9	0.9	64	98.8	15.8	753	78.9
9-H.W.	2	88.2	1.5	122	98.2	13.8	638	84.3
	3	93.7	1.9	161	98.0	17.3	754	81.5
10-W.G.	2	87.1	3.0	239	96.5	11.9	604	86.4
	3	78.1	3.4	289	95.6	12.0	534	84.7
	4	84.8	3.0	242	96.4	12.4	625	85.4
11-M.B.	3	89.7	1.4	125	98.4	12.0	682	86.6
	4	109.6	1.4	121	98.7	10.8	606	90.2
	5	119.7	1.7	129	98.6	9.8	480	91.8
Group mean		100.0	2.5	200	97.5	16.1	757	83.6
±SE		±3.86	±0.42	±32.8	±0.37	±1.08	±45.1	±1.03
Patients with mild renal failure—GFR 40—75 ml/min								
6-A.G.	2	52.5	1.4	130	97.3	12.5	623	76.2
	3	64.1	1.1	97	98.2	11.8	542	81.7
7-A.K.	2	73.7	1.4	110	98.2	9.9	682	86.6
8-B.P.	3	74.3	1.0	89	98.6	11.3	500	84.7
	4	68.1	1.0	78	98.6	9.6	440	85.9
9-H.W.	1	64.9	1.8	147	97.3	15.2	712	76.5
10-W.G.	1	47.5	4.0	259	91.5	4.1	223	91.4
11-M.B.	1	64.0	1.6	133	97.4	7.1	439	88.9
	2	66.4	2.7	206	96.0	9.9	456	85.1
12-B.L.	1	73.9	2.5	211	96.6	22.2	634	69.9
13-A.S.	1	54.4	1.3	108	97.6	7.9	483	85.5
	2	45.2	1.4	111	97.0	6.9	385	82.2
	3	58.4	0.9	77	98.5	7.1	384	87.8
Group mean		62.1	1.7	135	97.1	10.4	500	83.3
±SE		±2.72	±0.24	±10.7	±0.52	±1.27	±38.1	±1.65
Patients with moderate renal failure—GFR 20—40 ml/min								
14-Z.U.	1	23.6	1.6	128	93.2	11.4	700	51.9
15-J.W.	1	21.4	3.3	361	84.7	14.9	693	30.6
16-J.W.	1	28.3	1.9	141	93.3	6.7	300	76.3
Group mean		24.4	2.3	210	90.5	11.0	564	52.9
±SE		±2.03	±0.52	±75.6	±2.85	±2.37	±132.2	±13.20

Table 10 (continued)

Patient	Study	GFR ml/min	C_{Ca} ml/min	U_{Ca} mg/day	T_{Ca} %	C_{Pi} ml/min	U_{Pi} mg/day	T_{Pi} %
F		49.79	1.77	1.21	15.51	6.09	7.98	22.86
p		<0.001	NS	NS	<0.001	<0.01	<0.01	<0.001
Mean for all patients		80.6	2.1	178	96.8	13.7	651	81.0
±SE		±4.69	±0.27	±20.6	±0.46	±0.89	±36.1	±18.34

GFR = the true glomerular filtration rate of water; C_{Ca} and C_{Pi} = clearances, T_{Ca} and T_{Pi} = renal tubular reabsorptions, and U_{Ca} and U_{Pi} = urinary excretions of calcium and phosphate, respectively; F = the ratio from the between-subgroups variance estimate to the within-subgroups variance estimate; p = probability that an F-ratio from two variance estimates exceeds the tabulated critical values at a given level of confidence—values higher than 0.05 are nonsignificant (NS).

patients with mild renal failure, and 24.4 ± 2.03 ml/min in patients with moderate renal failure.

Calcium clearance was normal in all patients but one (case 4-F.S., 2nd study), in whom it was enormously raised. The analysis of variance did not show any significant difference between the subgroup means. The mean value for all patients was 2.1 ± 0.27 ml/min. The tubular reabsorption of calcium was reduced in one patient of the 1st subgroup (case 4-F.S., 2nd study), in one of the 2nd subgroup (case 10-W.G.), and in all patients of the 3rd subgroup. The means and variances of the first and second subgroup, 97.5 ± 0.37 per cent and 97.1 ± 0.52 per cent of the filtered calcium, respectively, did not differ significantly, but the mean and variance of the third subgroup, 90.5 ± 2.85 per cent, were significantly greater than those of the former two subgroups ($p < 0.001$). The mean value for all patients was 96.8 ± 0.46 per cent, which might suggest that the patients with plasmacytoma had normal tubular reabsorption, irrespective of renal damage. The tubular reabsorption of calcium paralleled the level of diffusible calcium in the plasma ultrafiltrate, according to the regression $y = 0.822 x + 0.84$ ($r = 0.923$; $p < 0.001$), where y is the tubular reabsorption of calcium in mg/100 ml filtrate, and x is the concentration of diffusible calcium in plasma ultrafiltrate in mg/100 ml (Fig. 38). It is worthy of note that the parallelism was poor in all patients with moderate renal failure and in one patient with mild renal failure. The non-reabsorbed part of the filtered calcium, that is, calcium excreted in urine, was equal to 178 ± 20.6 mg/day and did not show any significant difference between the subgroup means and variances. It was raised in two patients only (cases 4-F.S. and 15-J.W.). The daily urinary calcium paralleled the clearance of calcium, according to the regression $y = 0.0122 x$ ($r = 0.986$; $p < 0.001$), where y is the clearance of calcium in ml/min, and x is the urinary calcium in mg/day (Fig. 39). Only in one patient of the subgroup with moderate renal failure (case 15-J.W.) was the urinary excretion of calcium much greater than might have been suspected from calcium clearance.

Among the 16 patients, phosphate clearance was normal in ten, raised in five (in 6 studies), and reduced in one patient. The mean value for all patients was 13.7 ± 0.89 ml/min, but the analysis of variance showed significant differences be-

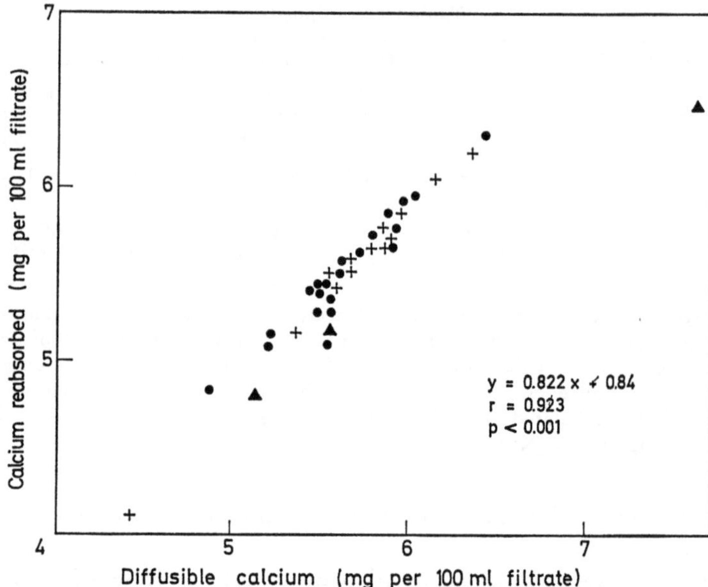

Fig. 38. The relation between tubular reabsorption of calcium per 100 ml filtrate and concentration of diffusible calcium per 100 ml ultrafiltrate in patients with plasmacytoma. ● designates patients with renal sufficiency; + with mild renal failure; ▲ with moderate renal failure

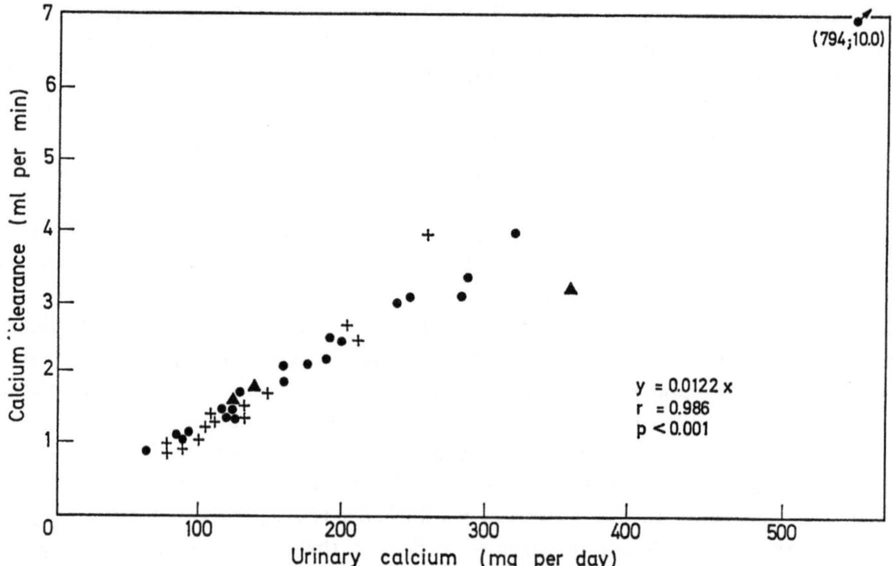

Fig. 39. The relation between calcium clearance and daily urinary calcium in patients with plasmacytoma. Designations as in Fig. 38

tween the subgroups (p < 0.01). The variances in each subgroup were almost the same, whereas the means differed significantly: the mean of the first subgroup, 16.1 ± 1.08 ml/min, differed from that of the second subgroup, 10.4 ± 1.27 ml/min,

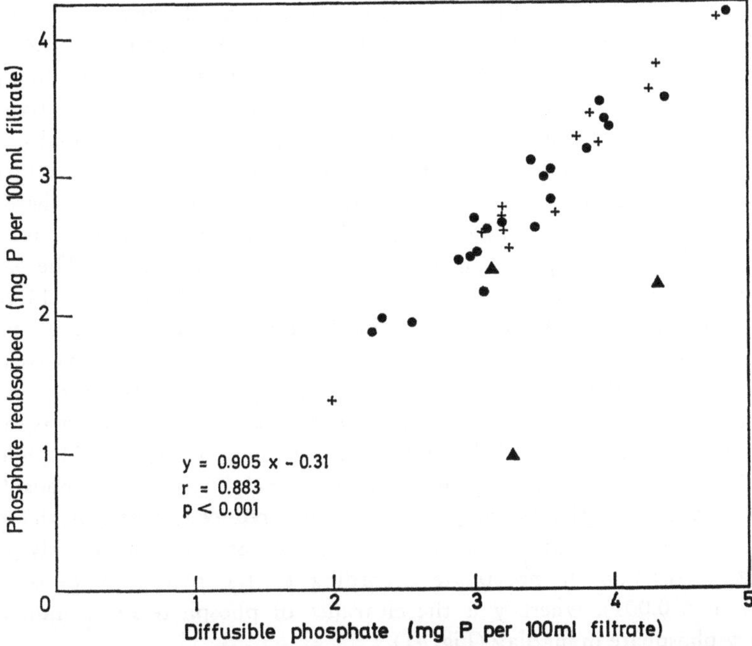

Fig. 40. The relation between tubular reabsorption of phosphate per 100 ml filtrate and concentration of diffusible phosphate per 100 ml ultrafiltrate in patients with plasmacytoma. ● designates patients with renal sufficiency; + with mild renal failure; ▲ with moderate renal failure

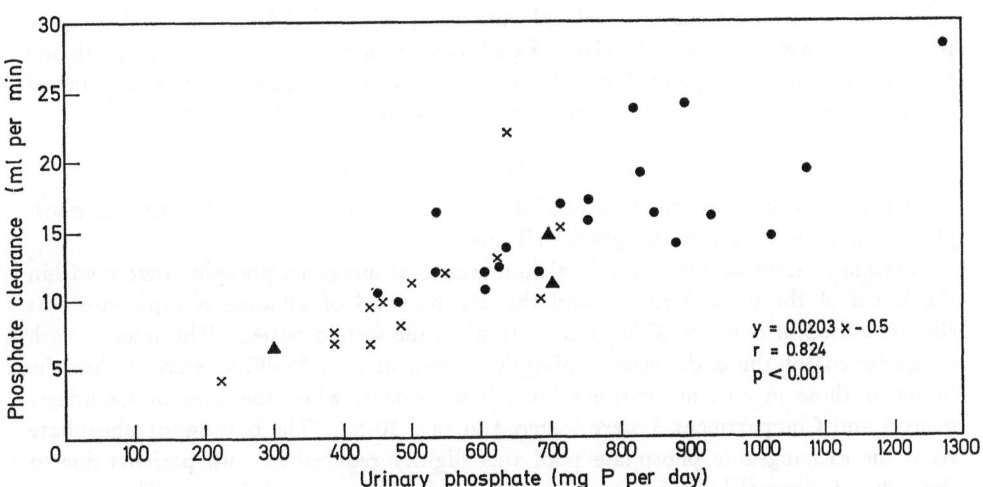

Fig. 41. The relation between phosphate clearance and daily urinary phosphate in patients with plasmacytoma. Designations as in Fig. 40

but not necessarily from that of the third subgroup, 11.0 ± 2.37 ml/min. The tubular reabsorption of phosphate was reduced in two patients of the 1st subgroup (cases 2-S.K. and 5-T.S., 1st study), in three patients of the 2nd subgroup (cases 6-A.G., second study, 9-H.W., first study, and 12-B.L.), and in all patients of the 3rd subgroup. The means and variances of the first and second subgroups, 83.6 ± 1.03 per cent and 83.3 ± 1.65 per cent, respectively, were almost the same, but the mean and variance of the third subgroup, 52.9 ± 13.20 per cent, were significantly different from those of the two former subgroups ($p < 0.001$). The tubular reabsorption of phosphate paralleled the level of diffusible phosphate in the plasma ultrafiltrate according to the regression $y = 0.905\, x - 0.31$ ($r = 0.883$; $p < 0.001$), where y is the tubular reabsorption of phosphate in mg/100 ml filtrate, and x is the concentration of diffusible phosphate in plasma ultrafiltrate in mg/100 ml (Fig. 40). The parallelism was poor only in two patients with moderate renal failure (cases 14-Z.U. and 15-J.W.). The non-reabsorbed part of the filtered phosphate, that is, phosphate excreted in urine, was equal to 651 ± 36.1 mg/day for all the patients treated as a whole. But the analysis of variance showed a difference among the subgroups ($p < 0.01$), and the studentized range test showed that this difference was due to the difference between the means of the first and second subgroup ($p < 0.01$), which were equal to 757 ± 45.1 and 500 ± 38.1 mg/day, respectively. The urinary phosphate was raised in 4 patients of the 1st subgroup only, and reduced in one of the 2nd subgroup and in another of the 3rd subgroup. The phosphate clearance strictly paralleled the urinary excretion of phosphate according to the regression $y = 0.0203 - 0.5$ ($r = 0.824$; $p < 0.001$), where y is the clearance of phosphate in ml/min, and x is the urinary phosphate in mg/day (Fig. 41).

Calcium Kinetics

The plasma data and the results of the compartmental analysis of calcium kinetics in 2 patients are given in Table 11.

Plasma concentrations of total calcium, total inorganic phosphate, and alkaline phosphatase were normal. The sizes of each compartment, mean outflows of calcium from the exchangeable pools, bone accretion rates, urinary excretion rates, and faecal excretions of endogenous calcium were within the limits of the normal range.

Inorganic Phosphate Kinetics

The plasma data and the results of the compartmental analysis of inorganic phosphate kinetics in 2 patients are given in Table 12.

Plasma concentrations of total calcium and total inorganic phosphate were within the limits of the normal range, and the plasma level of alkaline phosphatase was slightly raised in one (19-W.N.) and normal in the second patient. The sizes of each compartment of the exchangeable phosphate pool of case 19-W.N. were within the limits of those in patients without bone involvement, while the sizes of Compartment 1 and Compartment 3 were lowered in case 20-S.C. The outflow of phosphate from the exchangeable phosphate pool was slightly reduced in both patients due to the reduced internal loss and faecal excretion of endogenous phosphate. The urinary excretions of phosphate were normal in both patients.

The reduced internal loss might be due to the reduced bone accretion rate of inorganic phosphate. The rather low value of calcium accretion rate in both patients in whom the kinetics of calcium was studied (cases 17-B.P. and 18-A.S.), being taken as the basis for calculations, indicates that the mean value of 0.209 g Ca/m² per day has to be accompanied by 0.114 g P/m² per day, which is less than 12 per cent of the

Table 11. *Plasma values, compartment sizes, and flow constants of calcium*

Patient	Sex	Age	BSA	[Ca]$_P$	[P$_i$]$_P$	Alk. P'tase	Compartment sizes				Flow constants			
							1	2	3	Total	ϱ_{01}	V_0^+	V_u	V_f
		yrs	m²	mg/100 ml		K-A U			g/m²				g/day·m²	
17-P.B.	M	50	1.70	10.03	2.96	—	0.69	0.72	1.21	2.62	0.424	0.200	0.098	0.126
18-A.S.	F	49	1.63	9.36	3.01	11.2	0.66	0.47	0.75	1.88	0.412	0.235	0.093	0.084
Normal range														
Lowest							0.53	0.36	0.59	2.05	0.385	0.148	0.037	0.049
Highest							1.07	1.07	1.87	3.42	0.713	0.412	0.198	0.149

BSA = body surface area; [Ca]$_P$ = plasma concentration of total calcium; [P$_i$]$_P$ = plasma concentration of total inorganic phosphate; ϱ_{01} = the rate of unidirectional calcium loss; V_0^+ = the calcium accretion rate; V_u = the urinary calcium excretion rate; V_f = the faecal endogenous calcium excretion rate.

Table 12. *Plasma values, compartment sizes, and flow constants of inorganic phosphate*

Patient	Sex	Age	BSA	[Ca]$_P$	[P$_i$]$_P$	Alk. P'tase	Compartment sizes				Flow constants			
							1	2	3	Total	ϱ_{01}	ϱ_i	ϱ_u	ϱ_f
		yrs	m²	mg/100 ml		K-A U			g/m²				g/day·m²	
19-W.N.	M	33	1.71	9.58	3.30	16.3	0.43	0.96	7.90	9.29	1.089	0.640	0.398	0.051
20-S.C.	M	57	1.93	10.44	3.76	11.1	0.37	1.03	3.42	4.82	1.189	0.706	0.447	0.036
Normal range														
Lowest							0.44	0.69	5.43	7.14	1.247	0.808	0.367	0.058
Highest							0.78	1.75	10.38	11.93	1.594	1.074	0.531	0.088

BSA = body surface area; [Ca]$_P$ = plasma concentration of total calcium; [P$_i$]$_P$ = plasma concentration of total inorganic phosphate; ϱ_{01} = the rate of internal loss of phosphate; ϱ_u = the urinary phosphate excretion rate; ϱ_f = the faecal endogenous phosphate excretion rate.

total internal loss of phosphate. Since the normal value is at least 16 per cent, the lowered bone accretion rate of inorganic phosphate might be responsible for the low internal loss of phosphate.

2. Patients with Cancer of the Breast

2.1. Clinical Material

The material comprises 20 females with carcinoma of the breast. In 4 patients no apparent bone lesions, and in 16 patients multiple and widespread bone metastases were found. Among the 20 patients, the plasma state and renal handling of calcium and inorganic phosphate were studied in 6; these studies were repeated after oophorectomy in 3 patients. The kinetics of calcium metabolism has been studied in 12 other patients, and the kinetics of inorganic phosphate metabolism in the two remaining ones. The pertinent clinical data are presented in Table 13.

Table 13. *Clinical data on patients with breast cancer*

Patient	Age (yrs)	Stage [a]	Bones affected	Course of disease
1-A.R.	32	D	Pelvis	Regression
2-J.C.	45	D	Pelvis; r. rib 6	Progression
3-J.K.	49	D$_{BA}$	Pelvis; r. femur	Progression
4-H.K.	48	D	Pelvis; r. femur; skull	Regression
5-H.W.	41	D$_{BA}$	Pelvis; femurs; r. rib 4 and 12; l. rib 6; vert. Th 12	Regression
6-A.G.	45	D$_{BA}$	Pelvis; femurs; vert. L 1—L 4; ribs; skull	Progression
7-N.A.	49	D$_A$	Pelvis; r. rib 6	Progression
8-K.W.	51	D$_A$	Pelvis; vert. Th 11—L 1	Progression
9-R.S.	42	D$_A$	Pelvis; femurs; vert. L 1—L 4	Regression
10-J.A.	45	D$_A$	Pelvis; l. femur; ribs	Regression
11-J.R.	45	D$_A$	Pelvis; femurs; vert. Th 9—L 1	Progression
12-N.A.	55	D	None	Progression
13-W.W.	72	C	None	Stationary
14-D.J.	74	C	None	Stationary
15-S.J.	68	C	None	Stationary
16-K.J.	67	D	Pelvis; r. femur; vert. Th 3 and 11	Progression
17-P.J.	61	D	L. femur	Progression
18-K.J.	57	D	Pelvis; r. rib 8; vert. L 4	Progression
19-J.W.	58	D	Pelvis; r. rib 6; vert. L 1—L 3	Progression
20-K.S.	31	D$_A$	Pelvis; femurs; skull	Regression

[a] Classification after HAAGENSEN and COOLEY (1963). The subscripts BA are used to denote the study both before and after oophorectomy, and A to denote the study after oophorectomy only.

2.2. Results

Plasma State and Renal Handling of Calcium and Inorganic Phosphate

Observed data in 6 fertile-age patients and in 3 of these after oophorectomy are given in Tables 14 and 15. Statistical comparison was not made because the data were not normally distributed.

Table 14. *Indices of bone dynamics and plasma state of calcium and inorganic phosphate in patients with breast cancer*

Patient and study	Plasma Protein	Alk. P'tase	Urinary PP_i	$[Ca]_P$	$[Ca]_D$	Ca_{PB}		K_{CaProt}	$[P_i]_P$	$[P_i]_D$	P_{PB}
	g/100 ml	K-A U	mg/day	mg/100 ml		%	mg/g protein	M	mg/100 ml		%
Fertile patients											
1-A.R.$_1$	6.4	17.8	4.5	8.48	5.48	35.4	0.47	0.0129	3.00	2.29	23.5
2-J.C.$_1$	5.8	7.3	1.5	9.53	6.14	35.6	0.58	0.0135	3.17	2.74	13.6
3-J.K.$_1$	6.9	16.2	2.8	9.69	5.52	43.0	0.60	0.0098	2.60	2.22	14.4
4-H.K.$_1$	6.4	13.4	1.2	8.44	4.44	47.4	0.63	0.0076	4.06	3.49	14.1
5-H.W.$_1$	7.5	19.1	36.0	8.48	5.34	37.0	0.42	0.0142	3.80	3.16	16.9
6-A.G.$_1$	8.0	23.6	3.8	9.21	5.38	41.6	0.48	0.0124	3.80	3.22	15.3
Oophorectomized patients											
3-J.K.$_2$	6.9	9.2	2.7	9.68	5.54	42.8	0.60	0.0099	3.06	2.62	14.4
5-H.W.$_2$	6.7	32.1	2.2	8.37	5.19	38.0	0.47	0.0121	2.99	2.45	18.1
6-A.G.$_2$	8.4	16.8	2.4	10.48	6.08	42.0	0.52	0.0126	3.62	3.45	4.6
Normal range											
Lowest	6.2	4.0	0.3	8.80	5.40	37.0	0.44	0.0072	2.31	1.95	7.3
Highest	8.8	15.0	7.7	10.40	6.00	44.2	0.68	0.0150	4.47	3.81	22.9

PP_i = inorganic pyrophosphate; $[Ca]_P$ = plasma concentration of total calcium; $[Ca]_D$ = plasma concentration of diffusible calcium; Ca_{PB} = protein-bound plasma calcium; K_{CaProt} = dissociation constant of calcium proteinate; $[P_i]_P$ = plasma concentration of total inorganic phosphate; $[P_i]_D$ = plasma concentration of diffusible inorganic phasphate; P_{PB} = plasma protein-bound inorganic phosphate.

Of the six patients with advanced breast cancer, three (cases 1-A.R., 4-H.K. and 5-H.W.) showed an objective regression, that is, recalcification of osteolytic lesions, while the remaining three patients (cases 2-J.C., 3-J.K. and 6-A.G.) showed progression of bone lesions. Three patients were subjected to therapeutic oophorectomy: in two of them (cases 3-J.K. and 6-A.G.) further exacerbation was seen, and in one patient (case 5-H.W.) oophorectomy resulted in a striking regression, especially recalcification of bone lesions.

The plasma level of alkaline phosphatase was within the limits of the normal range in three patients, two fertile and one oophorectomized, and raised in the remainder. The excretion of urinary inorganic pyrophosphate was raised in one fertile patient, but it fell to a normal value after oophorectomy.

The plasma concentration of total calcium was below the inferior limit of the normal range in three patients with regressive cancer, and within the limits of the normal range in three patients with progressive cancer. After oophorectomy a trend towards depression of this concentration in one patient (case 5-H.W.), no significant change in one (case 3-J.K.), and a rise in another (case 6-A.G.) were observed.

The plasma concentration of diffusible calcium was significantly lowered in only one patient with regressive cancer (case 4-H.K.), slightly raised in another with progressive cancer (case 2-J.C.), and within the limits of the normal range in the remainder. After oophorectomy the changes paralleled those of total calcium, while the protein-bound calcium, being expressed as percentage of calcium bound, was essentially the same both before and after oophorectomy. Of the remaining three patients, the percentage of protein-bound calcium was slightly lowered in two (cases 1-A.R. and 2-J.C.) and slightly raised in one patient (case 4-H.K.). The amount of calcium bound with 1 gram of plasma protein and the dissociation constant of cal-

Table 15. *Renal handling of calcium and inorganic phosphate in patients with breast cancer*

Patient	Study	GFR ml/min	C_{Ca} ml/min	U_{Ca} mg/day	T_{Ca} %	C_{Pi} ml/min	U_{Pi} mg/day	T_{Pi} %
Fertile patients								
1-A.R.	1	24.7	1.1	84	95.7	12.8	493	48.1
2-J.C.	1	55.9	2.1	187	96.2	19.7	900	64.7
3-J.K.	1	67.6	3.1	250	95.3	14.6	546	78.4
4-H.K.	1	79.0	2.3	147	97.1	10.4	610	86.8
5-H.W.	1	78.8	2.6	201	96.7	6.1	327	92.2
6-A.G.	1	47.5	1.5	117	96.8	14.7	804	69.1
Oophorectomized patients								
3-J.K.	2	119.1	2.9	231	97.6	10.5	462	91.2
5-H.W.	2	85.6	0.8	59	99.1	14.3	587	83.3
6-A.G.	2	67.7	2.3	204	96.6	12.2	719	82.0
Normal range								
Lower		75.0	0.8	50	94.5	6.0	300	78.0
Highest		160.0	4.5	250	99.5	17.0	900	97.0

GFR = the true glomerular filtration rate of water; C_{Ca} and C_{Pi} = clearances, T_{Ca} and T_{Pi} = renal tubular reabsorptions, and U_{Ca} and U_{Pi} = urinary excretions of calcium and phosphate, respectively.

cium proteinate were within the limits of the normal range in all of the six patients. It indicates that the proteins of plasma, whose concentration was below the inferior limit of the normal range in only one patient with raised diffusible calcium (case 2-J.C.) and normal in the remainder, had a normal affinity for calcium.

The plasma concentration of both total and diffusible inorganic phosphate were within the limits of the normal range. The protein-binding of inorganic phosphate was essentially normal, being only insignificantly raised in one patient and lowered in another.

Renal sufficiency has been found in only two patients with regressive cancer (cases 4-H.K. and 5-H.W.), mild renal failure in three patients with progressive cancer (cases 2-J.C., 3-J.K. and 6-A.G.), and moderate renal failure in one patient with regressive cancer (case 1-A.R.). The true glomerular filtration rate increased after castration in all patients subjected to this therapy.

Calcium clearance, tubular reabsorption of calcium, and daily urinary calcium were within the limits of the normal range in all patients. But, in patient 5-H.W., the only case in whom after oophorectomy striking recalcification began, the clearance of calcium and the daily urinary calcium strikingly fell and the tubular reabsorption of calcium rose. In patient 6-A.G., in whom oophorectomy did not arrest exaggeration of the osteolytic process, the clearance of calcium as well as the urinary calcium rose, while the tubular reabsorption did not change.

Phosphate clearance was raised in only one patient and normal in the remainder. In three patients the tubular reabsorption of phosphate was reduced and paralleled the true glomerular filtration rate. Despite the disturbed reabsorption of filtered phosphate, the daily urinary phosphate was within the limits of the normal range in all patients.

Calcium Kinetics

The plasma data and the results of compartmental analysis of calcium kinetics in five oophorectomized patients and in seven post-menopausal patients have been given in Table 16 and Fig. 42 and 43.

Oophorectomized patients. — Of the 5 patients with advanced cancer of the breast, two (cases 9-R.S. and 10-J.A.) responded to oophorectomy and showed an objective regression, especially, recalcification of osteolytic lesions, whereas three (cases 7-N.A., 8-K.W. and 11-J.R.) after oophorectomy showed further rapid progression of cancer, especially further increase in the extent of bone lesions.

Plasma concentration of total calcium was normal in three (cases 7-N.A., 10-J.A. and 11-J.R.) and raised in two patients (cases 8-K.W. and 9-R.S.). All patients had normal plasma concentration of total inorganic phosphate, but showed a significant elevation of plasma alkaline phosphatase. In three patients (cases 7-N.A., 8-K.W. and 9-R.S.) the accretion rate tended to be elevated, but the pool sizes of the compartments were normal (Figs. 42 and 43). This elevated accretion rate was accompanied by hypercalciuria, moderate in one (case 7-N.A.) and high in the two patients with hypercalcaemia (cases 8-K.W. and 9-R.S.). In two patients (cases 10-J.A. and 11-J.R.) the accretion rate and the pool sizes of Compartment 2 and Compartment 3 were significantly raised. Daily urinary calcium was at the upper limit of the normal range in one (case 10-J.A.) and at the lower limit in another patient (case 11-J.R.).

Table 16. *Plasma values, compartment sizes, and flow constants of calcium in patients with breast cancer*

Patient	BSA	[Ca]$_P$	[P$_i$]$_P$	Alk. P'tase	Compartment sizes				Flow constants			
					1	2	3	Total	ϱ_{01}	V_0^+	V_u	V_f
	m^2	mg/100 ml		K-A U		g/m^2				g/m^2 per day		
Oophorectomized patients												
7-N.A	1.81	10.10	3.27	20.0	0.67	0.67	1.83	3.17	0.636	0.388	0.212	0.036
8-K.W.	1.78	11.70	3.25	19.2	1.11	1.01	1.72	3.84	0.877	0.462	0.337	0.078
9-R.S.	1.68	11.30	3.50	17.4	0.57	0.66	1.06	2.29	0.911	0.483	0.390	0.038
10-J.A.	1.59	9.47	3.20	27.4	1.23	1.68	3.03	5.94	1.374	1.160	0.152	0.062
11-J.R.	1.67	10.21	3.14	32.4	1.24	1.71	3.12	6.07	1.480	1.371	0.035	0.074
Postmenopausal patients												
12-N.A.	1.45	9.70	2.60	28.8	0.73	0.61	1.22	2.56	0.446	0.272	0.122	0.052
13-W.W.	1.80	9.70	3.17	9.0	0.58	1.08	1.36	3.02	0.440	0.212	0.189	0.039
14-D.J.	1.61	10.30	3.00	6.0	0.79	0.59	1.50	2.88	0.503	0.329	0.091	0.083
15-S.J.	1.87	9.81	2.00	3.4	0.68	0.75	1.16	2.59	0.609	0.474	0.052	0.083
16-K.J.	1.76	9.74	3.04	17.9	0.82	0.63	0.91	2.36	0.431	0.276	0.100	0.055
17-P.J.	1.52	10.55	3.02	18.8	1.06	1.05	1.73	3.84	0.727	0.514	0.107	0.106
18-K.J.	1.97	9.72	4.12	18.0	0.67	0.25	1.40	2.32	0.268	0.038	0.182	0.048
Normal range												
Lowest		8.80	2.31	4.0	0.53	0.36	0.59	2.05	0.385	0.148	0.037	0.049
Highest		10.40	4.47	15.0	1.07	1.07	1.87	3.42	0.713	0.412	0.198	0.149

BSA = body surface area; [Ca]$_P$ = plasma concentration of total calcium; [P$_i$]$_P$ = plasma concentration of total inorganic phosphate; ϱ_{01} = the rate of unidirectional loss of calcium; V_0^+ = the bone accretion rate of calcium; V_u = the urinary calcium excretion rate; V_f = the faecal endogenous calcium excretion rate.

SPRINGER-VERLAG
BERLIN · HEIDELBERG · NEW YORK

1 BERLIN 33
Heidelberger Platz 3 / *Telefon: Sammelnummer* 82 20 01
Berlin-West
Fernschreiber: 01 - 83 319

Redaktion / Editorial Board

Abt. VI, 30.6.1970 /Ja.

Radiologia Diagnostica

Wir senden Ihnen anbei ein Rezensionsexemplar unseres soeben erschienenen Werkes:
We have pleasure in sending you a review copy of our new book:

Recent Results in Cancer Research, <u>Vol.27</u>
Editor in chief: P. Rentchnick

SZYMENDERA, J., Institute of Oncology, Warsaw
<u>Bone Mineral Metabolism in Cancer</u>

43 fig. XI, 110 pages. 1970. Cloth DM 32,--; US $ 8.80

Berlin-Heidelberg-New York: Springer-Verlag (H)

<u>Title No. 3642</u>

und bitten Sie um eine baldige Besprechung in Ihrer Zeitschrift.
Please be so kind to publish the review including the bibliographical data in near future.

Wir bitten, **einen Besprechungsbeleg an unsere Abteilung VI** zu senden.
Please send **one cutting for the attention of our "Abteilung VI"**.

Hochachtungsvoll / Yours truly,

SPRINGER-VERLAG
Abteilung VI

<u>Anlage / Enclosure</u>

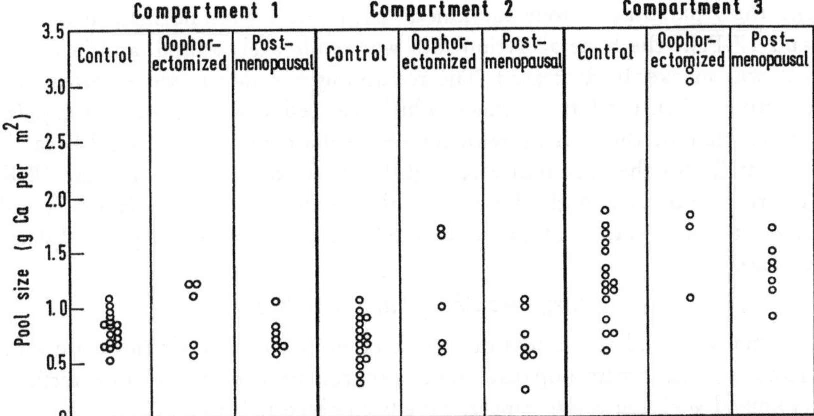

Fig. 42. The pool sizes of particular compartments of the exchangeable calcium pool in control cases, and in oophorectomized and postmenopausal patients with breast cancer

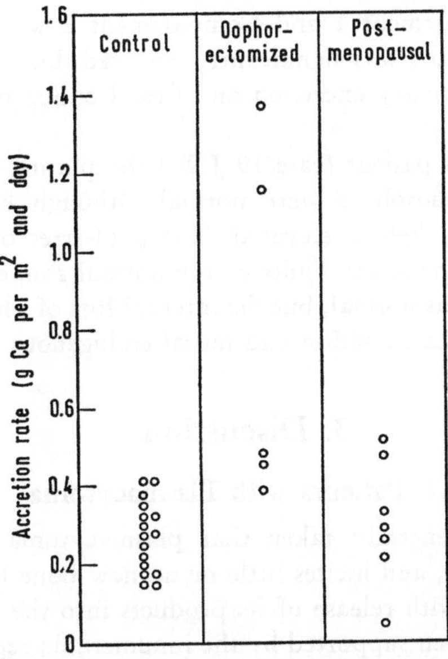

Fig. 43. The calcium accretion rates in control cases, and in oophorectomized and postmeno-pausal patients with breast cancer

Postmenopausal patients. — Of the 7 patients with advanced breast cancer, four were free from bone metastases and three showed rapid progression of disease and multiple osteolytic lesions.

Plasma concentration of total calcium was normal in all the patients but one, who showed a value slightly exceeding the upper limit of the normal range (case 17-P.J.). Plasma concentration of total inorganic phosphate was depressed in one (case 15-S.J.) and normal in the remaining patients. Plasma concentrations of alkaline phosphatase were normal in patients with stationary cancer of the breast (cases 13-W.W., 14-D.J. and 15-S.J.), and elevated in the remainder.

Among the 7 patients, in four the kinetic parameters were normal, in two (cases 15-S.J. and 17-P.J.) the bone accretion rate was moderately raised, and in one (case 18-K.J.) it was markedly decreased. The remaining parameters were normal except for Compartment 2 in the latter patient, which was reduced (Figs. 42 and 43). It has to be stressed that in the patient with hypophosphataemia (case 15-S.J.), calciuria was rather small and the accretion rate slightly elevated. One patient (case 18-K.J.) showed the reverse picture: high plasma phosphate concentration albeit not exceeding the upper limit of the normal range, moderate hypercalciuria, and a marked decrease of the accretion rate.

Inorganic Phosphate Kinetics

The plasma data and the results of compartmental analysis of phosphate kinetics in two patients, one postmenopausal with progressive cancer and one fertile-age, oophorectomized with regressive cancer, have been given in Table 17.

In the oophorectomized patient (case 20-K.S.) the plasma concentration of total calcium was at the high limit of the normal range, the concentration of total phosphate was normal, and the level of alkaline phosphatase was significantly elevated. The pool sizes of Compartment 1 and Compartment 2 were reduced. The rate of unidirectional phosphate loss was significantly elevated due to the rise in the rate of internal loss, while the urinary excretion and faecal endogenous excretion of phosphate were normal.

In the postmenopausal patient (case 19-J.W.) the plasma concentrations of total calcium and inorganic phosphate were normal although high, and the level of alkaline phosphatase was slightly elevated. The pool-sizes of Compartment 1 and Compartment 2 were at the lower limits of the normal range. The rate of unidirectional loss of phosphate was normal, but the internal loss of phosphate was depressed, while the urinary phosphate excretion and faecal endogenous excretion of phosphate were high.

3. Discussion

3.1. Patients with Plasmacytoma

The view has been generally taken that plasmacytoma results in widespread destruction of the skeleton, and incites little or no new bone formation. Hence, only osteolysis in conjunction with release of its products into the blood stream might be expected. This view has been supported by the innumerable reports on the occurrence of hypercalcaemia in about half the patients with plasmacytoma (APONTE, 1963; BENTZEL et al., 1964). Serum concentrations of calcium as high as 18.4 mg per 100 ml were seen (BENTZEL et al., 1964) despite usually normal concentrations of inorganic phosphate and alkaline phosphatase.

When strontium bone scanning became widely used for detection of metastatic cancer, positive bone scans were obtained also in plasmacytoma, indicating that reactive bone formation might be more common than was usually thought (CHARKES and SKLAROFF, 1965; CHARKES et al., 1966). If so, hypocalcaemia due to calcium accretion in newly formed bone matrix produced in reaction to tumour invasion should be seen, too.

Both hypercalcaemia and hypocalcaemia, and a whole range of values between the two extremes, have been found in the studied patients. The clinical material is

Table 17. *Plasma values, compartment sizes, and flow constants of inorganic phosphate in patients with breast cancer*

Patient	BSA	$[Ca]_P$	$[P_i]_P$	Alk. P'tase	Compartment sizes				Flow constants			
					1	2	3	Total	ϱ_{01}	ϱ_i	ϱ_u	ϱ_f
	m^2	mg/100 ml		K-A U		g/m^2				g/m^2 per day		
19-J.W.	1.65	10.30	4.44	19.8	0.40	0.62	6.58	7.60	1.382	0.651	0.547	0.184
20-K.S.	1.63	10.49	3.57	32.3	0.34	0.53	6.50	7.37	2.131	1.582	0.470	0.079
Normal range												
Lowest		8.80	2.31	4.0	0.44	0.69	5.43	7.14	1.247	0.808	0.367	0.058
Highest		10.40	4.47	15.0	0.78	1.75	10.38	11.93	1.594	1.074	0.531	0.088

BSA = body surface area; $[Ca]_P$ = plasma concentration of total calcium; $[P_i]_P$ = plasma concentration of total inorganic phosphate; ϱ_{01} = the rate of unidirectional phosphate loss; ϱ_i = the rate of internal loss of phosphate; ϱ_u = the urinary phosphate excretion rate; ϱ_f = the faecal endogenous phosphate excretion rate.

sufficient to ensure that the number of patients with hypercalcaemia in the plasma-cytoma group is no greater than that in other malignancies involving bone. WOODARD (1953) found hypercalcaemia in 8.4 per cent of 135 patients with miscellaneous tumours, excluding cancer of the breast and plasmacytoma. In the material presented, only two out of 20 patients, that is, 10 per cent, showed hypercalcaemia. But, slight hypocalcaemia was found in nearly the same percentage: in three out of 20 patients. The plasma concentration of diffusible calcium was raised in four and lowered in four other patients; neither state was stable but only a transient phenomenon during the course of the disease. A higher number of patients with raised diffusible calcium than with raised total calcium was found also by PRASAD and FLINK (1958). The lowered plasma concentration of diffusible calcium was accompanied by low daily urinary calcium in patients without any renal failure, and by slightly higher, near to the normal mean value, urinary calcium in patients with mild renal failure. Contrari-wise, the daily urinary calcium was increased only in patients with significantly raised plasma calcium.

These data seem indicate that increased osteolysis, releasing the products of resorbed bone into the blood stream and then into the urine, alternates with reversal of the osteolytic process and bone repair in the vicinity of neoplastic lesions. The latter increases demand on calcium and phosphate, which results in hypo-calcaemia and low calciuria. The wide variability in the plasma concentration of alkaline phosphatase and in urinary inorganic pyrophosphate suggests that both enhanced osteolysis and enhanced bone repair came into play in the patients in-vestigated.

The calcium-binding ability of plasma protein in patients with plasmacytoma had been shown to be markedly increased (RAWSON and SUNDERMAN, 1948). An abnormal affinity of plasma protein for calcium-binding has been found in about half the patients studied. But this affinity was both raised and reduced, with the latter predominating. This contradicts the findings of RAWSON and SUNDERMAN (1948), but agrees with more recent reports. WALSER (1962) found almost the same affinity of plasma protein for calcium-binding in normal subjects and in plasmacytoma patients with hypercalcaemia, although the variability in the latter group was much greater. DALE and KELLERMAN (1967) found reduced affinity in two and normal in three patients with plasmacytoma; and SMARSZ and ADAMSKI (1967) reported normal affinity in two and raised in three patients with plasmacytoma. The concentration of plasma protein was slightly lowered in four patients and increased in four others, although the means were almost the same.

The plasma concentrations of total and diffusible phosphate were not different from those of normal subjects, which is in agreement with the previous reports (APONTE, 1963). The percentage of plasma inorganic phosphate bound to protein was lower than that in the normal group, indicating the lower phosphate-binding ability of plasma protein, similar to that for calcium.

Renal involvement occurs quite often in plasmacytoma, due chiefly to obstruction of the tubules by casts of protein (APONTE, 1963). Among the 16 patients, mild renal failure was found in about half and moderate in 3 others. The mild renal failure showed a trend towards regression in only 3 patients. Calcium clearance was normal in all patients but one. A slightly reduced tubular reabsorption of cal-cium was found in all patients with moderate renal failure and in one without renal failure. The tubular reabsorption of calcium paralleled the plasma level of diffusible calcium, except in the above-mentioned patients. These observations are in agreement with those of Friis et al. (1968) who stated that tubular reabsorption did not change until the creatinine clearance fell below 40 ml/min.

Much greater variability was found in phosphate clearance. The greatest clearances were seen in patients without renal failure, and relatively low ones in patients with moderate renal failure. The tubular reabsorption of phosphate paralleled the level of diffusible phosphate in all but two patients with moderate renal failure. It has to be stressed that the percentage of tubular reabsorption of phosphate was reduced in two patients of the subgroup with renal sufficiency, in three patients of the subgroup with mild renal failure, and in all patients of the subgroup with moderate renal failure. If the relation between tubular reabsorption and plasma diffusible phosphate were not taken into consideration, an apparently lower tubular reabsorption would be seen in patients with higher concentrations of diffusible phosphate.

The kinetics of calcium metabolism in two patients with plasmacytoma and normocalcaemia showed that bone accretion rates and compartment sizes were relatively low, albeit within the normal range. It is in agreement with the data of Bentzel et al. (1964) and Myers et al. (1968) who found normal accretion rates and slightly lowered pool sizes of exchangeable calcium in normocalcaemic plasmacytoma patients. On the other hand, Bentzel et al. found in hypercalcaemic plasmacytoma patients elevated pools of exchangeable calcium, elevated accretion and resorption rates, and hypercalciuria; and Myers et al. found that hypercalcaemia was attended by an enhanced rate of accretion and resorption, the latter increased even more than the former.

The kinetics of inorganic phosphate metabolism roughly paralleled that of calcium: the internal loss of phosphate was slightly reduced, presumably due to the lowered demand on phosphate from bone. In one patient also Compartment 1 and Compartment 3 were reduced, presumably due to the reduced shares of bone in each.

The data presented above indicate that the plasma state, renal handling, and kinetics of metabolism of calcium and inorganic phosphate reflect the predominance of either the osteolysis or the remodelling of involved bone. It might be assumed that a slow progress of the disease favours the establishment of equilibrium at slightly reduced accretion rates and compartment sizes of calcium and inorganic phosphate. A rapid progress of plasmacytoma, and sometimes its arrest in response to therapy, may disturb this equilibrium, as reflected by either hypercalcaemia and hypercalciuria or hypocalcaemia and low calciuria, respectively. The former phenomenon is well known, whereas the latter has been overlooked heretofore.

3.2. Patients with Cancer of the Breast

Recently, Furth (1968) in his excellent lecture on Hormones and Neoplasia outlined the interrelation of hormones and breast cancer, which in epitome is the following:

In mammary tumour hormonal factors are indispensable components in carcinogenesis and control. The pituitary cell with mammotropic properties plays a determining role in inducing mammary tumours by carcinogens and their further control.

The evidence thus far points to prolactin as the specific mammary gland stimulant, while oestrogens act indirectly by stimulation of the pituitary acidophiles. Hence, for prophylaxis and control of hormone-responsive mammary tumours, procedures are needed to block mammotropin production and release by the pituitary. This is obtained by removing either the organ whis secretes mammotropin (ablation or radiological destruction of pituitary) or the organ which acts indirectly (oophorectomy, alone or combined with adrenalectomy). In human breast cancer both interventions give about the same results.

The disturbances in the plasma state, renal handling, and kinetics of calcium metabolism have been seen as the result of the extent and activity of bone metastases per se (COREY et al., 1961; COREY et al., 1962; MYERS et al., 1966; MYERS et al., 1968), and as the effect of the production of an osteolytic sterol by breast cancer itself (GORDAN et al., 1966; GORDAN, 1967). Several facts appear to argue against the hypothesis that disturbances in the calcium metabolism are simply due to the simultaneous osteolysis: from bone infiltration by the tumour and from the action of osteolytic sterol.

Hypercalcaemia would be more frequent if only these two factors were responsible for bone mineral disturbances. WOODARD (1953) found hypercalcaemia in 9.4 per cent of 445 patients with breast cancer. BAKER (1956) reported hypercalcaemia in 10 per cent of untreated, and in 20 per cent of sex-hormone treated patients. HORTON and OLSON (1964) found hypercalcaemia in 13 per cent of 126 patients. It has to be stressed that hypercalcaemia was not associated with a more severe or rapidly progressive form of the disease (HORTON and OLSON, 1964). On a specific hormone therapy, hypercalcaemia returns to or towards normocalcaemia or, contrariwise, it either appears or increases simultaneously with altered activity of the cancer cells (HERRMAN et al., 1949; KENNEDY et al., 1953; PERSSON et al., 1954; KENNEDY et al., 1955).

These observations indicate that the alterations in calcium metabolism might be better explained by taking into account the hormonal influences. A trial of such an interpretation was presented in a previous paper (SZYMENDERA et al., 1967 a). Further investigations and FURTH's theory now permit better interpretation of the experimental data obtained.

Significant hypercalcaemia was found in two of the 20 patients (10 per cent), and values on the upper borderline were found in 3 others. But, a slight hypocalcaemia was also found in 3 patients. Hypercalcaemia was accompanied by hypercalciuria, and the upper borderline calcaemia by moderate calciuria. In the 3 patients with hypocalcaemia, plasma concentration of diffusible calcium was normal in two and decreased in only one patient, in whom low calciuria was observed. It is worth remembering that the patients with hypocalcaemia were in the stage of regression; while of the two patients with hypercalcaemia one was in the stage of regression and one in that of progression. Of the 3 patients with values of total calcium on the upper borderline, one was in the stage of regression, and two had progressive cancer.

Of the 3 patients subjected to castration, only one showed a striking regression after that intervention. It was accompanied by a fall in plasma and urinary calcium. In one patient castration was without any apparent effect, and in the remaining one oophorectomy did not arrest the rapidly progressive cancer. Plasma and urinary calcium did not change in the former and rose in the latter patient. Since only oophorectomy was performed in these patients, it might be possible that vicarious secretion of oestrogens by the adrenals further stimulated the pituitary acidophiles, and hence oestolysis from direct bone destruction by metastases and from osteolytic sterol came into play.

Kinetic studies in postmenopausal patients indicate that the fall in oestrogens (PROCOPÉ, 1969) might diminish the stimulation of pituitary acidophiles, which in turn might diminish the progress of cancer. Hence, the metabolic calcium parameters were essentially within the limits of the normal range, except for one patient who showed marked decrease of the accretion rate.

Surgical castration causes a rapid and complete cessation of ovarian function (BLOCK et al., 1958; LEWISON, 1965; NISSEN-MAYER and SANNER, 1963 a and b; PERSSON and RISHOLM, 1964; PROCOPÉ, 1969) and in turn stimulates the adrenal glands (PERSSON and RISHOLM, 1964). However, the role of the adrenals in vicarious secretion of oestrogens is known to vary quantitatively and qualitatively from patient to patient (LEWISON, 1965; PROCOPÉ, 1969). When the vicarious secretion of oestrogens by the adrenals is low, which in turn diminishes the stimulation of the pituitary acidophiles, control of the tumour is combined with recalcification of bone osteolytic lesions, which enhances the accretion rate and decreases plasma and urinary calcium. When the vicarious secretion of oestrogens by the adrenals replaces those that had been secreted by the intact ovaries, hypercalcaemia and hypercalciuria persist; the accretion rate may be slightly enhanced, but an even greater increase is observed in resorption rate (MYERS et al., 1968).

The same trends were observed in the kinetics of inorganic phosphate metabolism: high internal loss and normal urinary phosphate in oophorectomized patients with regressive cancer, and low internal loss and high urinary phosphate in progressive breast cancer.

The data presented here seem to indicate that the simultaneous osteolysis from bone infiltration by neoplasma and from production of an oesteolytic sterol by the tumour itself, as well as the indirect influence of oestrogens produced by either ovaries or adrenals, have to be taken into account when interpreting the changes in plasma state, renal handling, and kinetics of metabolism of calcium and phosphate in patients with cancer of the breast.

General Summary

Chapter 1. Bone as a tissue is composed of cells, organic matric and mineral. Bone cells stem from the preosteoblast. Organic matrix consists of collagen and ground substance. Bone mineral contains two major phases: amorphous calcium phosphate and crystalline bone apatite.

Chapter 2. The clinical approach to bone tissue metabolism depends on studying the plasma state, renal handling, balance, and kinectics of calcium and inorganic phosphate. The latter may be investigated by the aid of tracers and analyzed by compartmental analysis.

Chapter 3. The plasma state and renal handling of calcium and inorganic phosphate were studied under controlled metabolic conditions. The kinetics of calcium was studied by the aid of ^{45}Ca and ^{47}Ca, and that of inorganic phosphate by the aid of ^{32}P. A three-compartment parallel open system model was used for data analysis.

Chapter 4. The majority of patients without bone secondaries had normal plasma state, renal handling, and kinetics of calcium and phosphate, although the variability of each parameter was greater than in normal subjects.

Fertile-age women showed normal remodelling of bone, but the combined curie and X-ray therapy of cancer of the uterine cervix was, in these women, a factor triggering the development of osteoporosis.

Chapter 5. In plasmacytoma patients, the plasma state, renal handling, and kinetics of calcium and phosphate reflected only the osteolytic and remodelling processes.

In patients with cancer of the breast, the simultaneous osteolysis from bone infiltration by neoplasma and from osteolytic sterol produced by the tumour itself, as well as the stimulation of pituitary mammotropic cells by oestrogens, influence the metabolic parameters of calcium and phosphate.

Appendix

An Analytical Solution of the Parallel Three-Compartment Open System Model

Notations

M_i — amount of substance in compartment i of the exchangeable system, in grams;

λ_{ij} — fractional rate constant of substance transferred into compartment i from compartment j per unit time, in fraction per day;

$\varrho_{ij} = \lambda_{ij} M_j$ — intercompartmental flow constant of substance transferred into compartment i from compartment j, in grams per day;

C_i — specific activity of substance in the ith compartment, in fraction of the tracer dose per gram of substance;

A_{ij} — coefficient of the jth exponential term of the specific activity curve in the ith compartment, in fraction of the tracer dose per gram of substance;

α_j — exponential constant in the jth exponential term, in fraction per day.

Analysis

The steady-state parallel three-compartment open system model, presented in Fig. 27, is adequately characterized by a complete set of the fractional rate constants λ_{ij}, and the compartment sizes M_j. The following set of simultaneous first-order differential equations describes the behaviour of the specific activity of calcium or phosphate in particular compartments of the exchangeable system

$$\frac{dC_1}{dt} = -(\lambda_{21} + \lambda_{31} + \lambda_{01})\, C_1 + \lambda_{21}\, C_2 + \lambda_{31}\, C_3$$

$$\frac{dC_2}{dt} = \lambda_{12}\, C_1 - \lambda_{12}\, C_2 \qquad\qquad (1)$$

$$\frac{dC_3}{dt} = \lambda_{13}\, C_1 - \lambda_{13}\, C_3 \,.$$

The successive elimination of variables C_1 and C_3 from this set leads to the following third-order differential equation with respect to C_2

$$\frac{d^3C_2}{dt^3} + (\lambda_{21}+\lambda_{31}+\lambda_{01}+\lambda_{12}+\lambda_{13})\frac{d^2C_2}{dt^2} + \{\lambda_{13}(\lambda_{21}+\lambda_{01}+\lambda_{12}) + \lambda_{12}(\lambda_{31}+\lambda_{01})\}\frac{dC_2}{dt} + \lambda_{01}\lambda_{12}\lambda_{13} = 0 . \tag{2}$$

The characteristic equation of relation (2) is

$$\alpha^3 + (\lambda_{21}+\lambda_{31}+\lambda_{01}+\lambda_{12}+\lambda_{13})\,\alpha^2 + \{\lambda_{13}(\lambda_{21}+\lambda_{01}+\lambda_{12}) + \lambda_{12}(\lambda_{31}+\lambda_{01})\}\,\alpha + \lambda_{01}\lambda_{12}\lambda_{13} = 0 . \tag{3}$$

The roots of this characteristic equation α_i, $i = 1$, 2 and 3, fulfil the following relations

$$\begin{aligned}
\alpha_1 + \alpha_2 + \alpha_3 &= -(\lambda_{21}+\lambda_{31}+\lambda_{01}+\lambda_{12}+\lambda_{13}) \\
\alpha_1\alpha_2 + \alpha_1\alpha_3 + \alpha_2\alpha_3 &= \{\lambda_{13}(\lambda_{21}+\lambda_{01}+\lambda_{12}) + \lambda_{12}(\lambda_{31}+\lambda_{01})\} \\
\alpha_1\alpha_2\alpha_3 &= -\lambda_{01}\lambda_{12}\lambda_{13} .
\end{aligned} \tag{4}$$

Hence, the general solution of the initial set (1) is given by

$$\begin{aligned}
C_2 &= \sum_{i=1}^{3} K_i \exp \alpha_i t \\
C_1 &= \sum_{i=1}^{3} K_i \frac{\alpha_i+\lambda_{12}}{\lambda_{12}} \exp \alpha_i t \\
C_3 &= \sum_{i=1}^{3} K_i \frac{\alpha_i(\alpha_i+\lambda_{21}+\lambda_{31}+\lambda_{01}+\lambda_{12})+\lambda_{12}(\lambda_{31}+\lambda_{01})}{\lambda_{31}\lambda_{12}} \exp \alpha_i t
\end{aligned} \tag{5}$$

where K_i, $i = 1$, 2 and 3, are the integration constants to be determined from the initial conditions.

The latter for $t = 0$ are as follows

$$\begin{aligned}
\sum_{i=1}^{3} K_i \frac{\alpha_i+\lambda_{12}}{\lambda_{12}} &= A_{11} + A_{12} + A_{13} \\
\sum_{i=1}^{3} K_i &= 0 \\
\sum_{i=1}^{3} K_i \frac{\alpha_i(\alpha_i+\lambda_{21}+\lambda_{31}+\lambda_{01}+\lambda_{12})+\lambda_{12}(\lambda_{31}+\lambda_{01})}{\lambda_{31}\lambda_{12}} &= 0 .
\end{aligned} \tag{6}$$

Knowing the integration constants K_i, one can form a set of three linear equations with respect to the model parameters λ_{ij}

$$\begin{aligned}
A_{11} &= \frac{2C_{10}(\alpha_1+\lambda_{12})}{(\alpha_2-\alpha_3)^2}\left(\alpha_1 + \frac{\alpha_2}{2} + \frac{\alpha_3}{2} + \lambda_{21}+\lambda_{31}+\lambda_{01}+\lambda_{12}\right) \\
A_{12} &= -\frac{C_{10}(\alpha_2+\lambda_{12})}{(\alpha_2-\alpha_1)(\alpha_2-\alpha_3)}(\alpha_1+\alpha_3+\lambda_{21}+\lambda_{31}+\lambda_{01}+\lambda_{12}) \\
A_{13} &= -\frac{C_{10}(\alpha_3+\lambda_{12})}{(\alpha_3-\alpha_1)(\alpha_3-\alpha_2)}(\alpha_1+\alpha_2+\lambda_{21}-\lambda_{31}+\lambda_{01}+\lambda_{12}) .
\end{aligned} \tag{7}$$

From expressions (7) and (4) the fractional rate constants are finally obtained. To simplify the notation, let

$$\begin{aligned}
P &= -\{\alpha_1(A_{12}+A_{13}) + \alpha_2(A_{11}+A_{13}) + \alpha_3(A_{11}+A_{12})\} \\
N &= A_{11}\alpha_2\alpha_3 + A_{12}\alpha_1\alpha_3 + A_{13}\alpha_1\alpha_2
\end{aligned}$$

and in these terms the corresponding λ_{ij} can be rewritten as

$$\lambda_{12} = \frac{P + \sqrt{P^2 - 4\,NC_{10}}}{2\,C_{10}} \tag{8}$$

$$\lambda_{13} = \frac{A_{12}\,(\alpha_2 - \alpha_1)\,(\alpha_2 - \alpha_3)}{C_{10}\,(\alpha_2 + \lambda_{12})} - \alpha_2 \tag{9}$$

$$\lambda_{01} = \frac{\alpha_1\,\alpha_2\,\alpha_3}{\lambda_{12}\,\lambda_{13}} \tag{10}$$

$$\lambda_{31} = \frac{\lambda_{13}\,(\alpha_1 + \alpha_2 + \alpha_3 + \lambda_{13}) + (\alpha_1\,\alpha_2 + \alpha_1\,\alpha_3 + \alpha_2\,\alpha_3) - \lambda_{12}\,\lambda_{01}}{\lambda_{12} - \lambda_{13}} \tag{11}$$

$$\lambda_{21} = -(\alpha_1 + \alpha_2 + \alpha_3 + \lambda_{31} + \lambda_{01} + \lambda_{12} + \lambda_{13})\,. \tag{12}$$

It should be stressed that in expressions (8)—(12) the signed values of α_i must be substituted. The specific activity of calcium or phosphate in Compartment 1 at zero time C_{10} follows from equation (6)

$$C_{10} = A_{11} + A_{12} + A_{13}\,. \tag{13}$$

The compartment sizes of the exchangeable system are given by

$$M_1 = 1/C_{10}; \quad M_2 = \varrho_{12}/\lambda_{12}; \quad M_3 = \varrho_{13}/\lambda_{13} \tag{14}$$

and the flow constants by

$$\varrho_{21} = \varrho_{12} = \lambda_{21}\,M_1; \quad \varrho_{31} = \varrho_{13} = \lambda_{31}\,M_1; \quad \varrho_{01} = \lambda_{01}\,M_1\,. \tag{15}$$

References

ADAMSON, L. F., ANAST, C. S.: Amino acid, potassium, and sulfate transport and incorporation by embryonic chick cartilage: The mechanism of the stimulatory effects of serum. Biochim. biophys. Acta (Amst.) 121, 10 (1966).

ALBRIGHT, F., SMITH, P. H., RICHARDSON, A. M.: Post-menopausal osteoporosis; its clinical features. J. Amer. med. Ass. 116, 2465 (1941).

ANAST, C., ARNAUD, C. D., RASMUSSEN, H., TENENHOUSE, A.: Thyrocalcitonin and the response to parathyroid hormone. J. clin. Invest. 46, 57 (1967).

ANNINO, J. S., RELMAN, A. S.: The effect of eating on some of the clinically important chemical constituents of the blood. Amer. J. clin. Path. 31, 155 (1959).

APONTE, G. E.: Nephrocalcinosis and nephrolithiasis in hyperparathyroidism. In: Evaluation of Thyroid and Parathyroid Functions. Eds.: F. W. SUNDERMAN and F. W. SUNDERMAN, JR. Philadelphia-Montreal: J. B. Lippincott Company 1963, p. 256.

ARNAUD, C., RASMUSSEN, H., ANAST, C.: Further studies on the interrelationship between parathyroid hormone and vitamin D. J. clin. Invest. 45, 1955 (1966).

AUBERT, J.-P., MILHAUD, G.: Méthode de mesure des principales voies du métabolisme calcique chez l'homme. Biochim. biophys. Acta (Amst.) 39, 122 (1960).

AVIOLI, L. V., BERMAN, M.: Mg^{28} kinetics in man. J. appl. Physiol. 21, 1688 (1966).

—, HENNEMAN, P. H.: Isotopic (Ca^{47}) analysis of the suppressive action of aspirin on Paget's disease of bone. In: Dynamic Studies of Metabolic Bone Disease. Eds.: O. H. PEARSON and G. F. JOPLIN. Oxford: Blackwell Scientific Publications 1964, p. 185.

— — Urinary pyrophosphate in disorders of bone metabolism. In: Calcified Tissues 1965. Eds.: H. FLEISCH, H. J. J. BLACKWOOD, and M. OWEN. Berlin-Heidelberg: Springer 1966, p. 67.

—, McDONALD, J. E., HENNEMAN, P. H., LEE, S. W.: The relationship of parathyroid activity to pyrophosphate excretion. J. clin. Invest. 45, 1093 (1966).

— —, SINGER, R. A.: Excretion of pyrophosphate in disorders of bone metabolism. J. clin. Endocr. 25, 912 (1965).

AVIOLI, L. V., PROCKOP, D. J.: Collagen degradation and the response to parathyroid extract in the intact rhesus monkey. J. clin. Invest. **46**, 217 (1967).

BAKER, W. H.: Abnormalities in calcium metabolism in malignancy; effects of hormone therapy. Amer. J. Med. **21**, 714 (1956).

BARRETT, A. J.: Cartilage. In: Comprehensive Biochemistry, v. 26-B. Eds. : M. FLORKIN and E. H. STOTZ. Amsterdam: Elesevier 1968, p. 425.

BAUD, C. A.: The fine structure of normal and parathormone-treated bone cells. In: Fourth European Symposium on Calcified Tissues. Eds.: P. J. GAILLARD, A. VAN DEN HOOFF, and R. STEENDIJK. Amsterdam: Excerpta Medica Foundation 1966, p. 4.

BAUER, G. C. H., CARLSSON, A., LINDQUIST, B.: Evaluation of accretion, resorption, and exchange reactions in the skeleton. Kgl. Fysiogr. Sallsk. i Lund Forh. **25**, 1 (1955).

— — — Metabolism and homeostatic function of bone. In: Mineral Metabolism, v. 1-A. Eds.: C. L. COMAR and F. BRONNER. New York-London: Academic Press 1961, p. 609.

BEAR, R. S.: The structure of collagen fibrils. Advanc. Protein Chem. **7**, 69 (1952).

BENOWITZ, N. L., TEREPKA, A. R.: Calcium binding to phosphoprotein in estrogenized rooster plasma studied by density-gradient centrifugation. Proc. Soc. exp. Biol. (N. Y.) **129**, 46 (1968).

BENTZEL, C. J., CARBONE, P. P., ROSENBERG, L.: The effect of prednisone on calcium metabolism and Ca^{47} kinetics in patients with multiple myeloma and hypercalcemia. J. clin. Invest. **43**, 2132 (1964).

BERKOWITZ, J. M., SHERMAN, J. L., JR., HART, H. E.: The rate of decarboxylation of mevalonic acid-l-C^{14} in man. Ann. N. Y. Acad. Sci. **108**, 250 (1963).

BERMAN, M.: Mathematical principles. In: Combined Clinical Staff Conference at the National Institutes of Health: The application of multicompartment analysis to problems of clinical medicine. Ann. intern. Med. **68**, 423 (1968).

BERNSTEIN, D., KLEEMAN, C. R., MAXWELL, M. H.: The effect of calcium infusions, parathyroid hormone, and vitamin D on renal clearance of calcium. Proc. Soc. exp. Biol. (N. Y.) **112**, 353 (1963).

BERSON, S. A., YALOW, R. S.: Parathyroid hormone in plasma in adenomatous hyperparathyroidism, uremia, and bronchogenic carcinoma. Science **154**, 907 (1966).

BETT, I. M., FRASER, G. P.: A rapid micro-method for determining serum calcium. Clin. chim. Acta **4**, 346 (1959).

BHATNAGAR, R. S., PROCKOP, D. J.: Dissociation of the synthesis of sulphated mucopolysaccharides and the synthesis of collagen in embryonic cartilage. Biochim. biophys. Acta (Amst.) **130**, 383 (1966).

—, ROSENBLOOM, J., KIVIRIKKO, K. I., PROCKOP, D. J.: Effect of cycloheximide on collagen biosynthesis as evidence for a postribosomal site for the hydroxylation of proline. Biochim. biophys. Acta (Amst.) **149**, 273 (1967).

BLOCK, G. E., VIAL, A. B., PULLEN, F. W.: Estrogen excretion following operative and irradiation castration in cases of mammary cancer. A preliminary report. Surgery **43**, 415 (1958).

BORNSTEIN, P.: The incomplete hydroxylation of individual prolyl residues in collagen. J. biol. Chem. **242**, 2572 (1967).

—, PIEZ, K. A.: A biochemical study of human skin collagen and the relation between intra- and intermolecular cross-linking. J. clin. Invest. **43**, 1813 (1964).

— — Collagen: Structural studies based on the cleavage of methionyl bonds. Science **148**, 1353 (1965).

BRONNER, F., RICHELLE, L. J., SAVILLE, P. D., NICHOLAS, J. A., COBB, J. R.: Quantitation of calcium metabolism in postmenopausal osteoporosis and in scoliosis. J. clin. Invest. **42**, 898 (1963).

—, SAVILLE, P. D., NICHOLAS, J. A., COBB, J. R., WILSON, P. D., JR., WILSON, P. D.: Calcium metabolism in man. Quantitation of calcium absorption and the excretion index. In: Radioisotopes and Bone. Eds.: F. C. McLEAN, P. LACROIX, and A. M. BUDY. Oxford: Blackwell Scientific Publications 1962, p. 17.

BROWNELL, G. L., BERMAN, M., ROBERTSON, J. S.: Nomenclature for tracer kinetics. Int. J. appl. Radiat. **19**, 249 (1968).

96 References

BURLEY, R. W.: Transphosphorylation of adenosine di- and triphosphates in the presence of calcium phosphate precipitates. Nature 208, 683 (1965).
CARE, A. D., KEYNES, W. M.: The role of parathyroid hormones in the absorption of calcium and magnesium from the small intestine. Proc. roy. Soc. Med. 57, 867 (1964).
CARLSSON, A.: Metabolism of radiocalcium in relation to calcium intake in young rats. Acta Pharmacol. Toxicol. 7, Suppl. 1 (1951).
CARROLL, E., PECHET, M.: Stimulation of bone formation by inorganic phosphate and inhibition of bone resorption by thyrocalcitonin. J. clin. Invest. (Abstr.) 46, 1043 (1967).
CESSI, C., BERNARDI, G.: The kinetics of enzymatic degradation and the structure of protein-polysaccharide complexes of cartilage. In: Structure and Function of Connective and Skeletal Tissue. Eds.: S. FITTON JACKSON, R. D. HARKNESS, S. M. PARTRIDGE, and G. R. TRISTRAM. London: Butterworths 1965, p. 152.
CHARKES, N. D., SKLAROFF, D. M.: Detection of occult metastases to bone by photoscanning with radioisotopes of strontium. In: Progress in Clinical Cancer, Vol. I. Ed.: I. ARIEL. New York: Grune & Stratton 1965, p. 235.
— — YOUNG, I.: A critical analysis of strontium bone scanning for detection of metastatic cancer. Amer. J. Roentgenol. 96, 647 (1966).
CHEN, P. S., TORIBARA, T. Y., WARNER, H.: Microdetermination of phosphorus. Analyt. Biochem. 28, 1756 (1956).
COHN, S. H., BOZZO, S. R., JESSEPH, J. E., CONSTANTINIDES, C., HUENE, D. R., GUSMANO, E. A.: Formulation and testing of a compartmental model for calcium metabolism in man. Radiat. Res. 26, (1965).
—, GUSMANO, E. A.: Kinetics of strontium and calcium skeletal metabolism in the rat. Proc. Soc. exp. Biol. (N. Y.) 126, 79 (1967).
—, LIPPINCOTT, S. W., GUSMANO, E. A., ROBERTSON, J. S.: Comparative kinetics of Ca^{47} and Sr^{85} in man. Radiat. Res. 19, 104 (1963).
COREY, K. R., KENNY, P., GREENBERG, E., LAUGHLIN, J. S.: Results of kinetic analysis and calcium balance studies in malignancy. In: Technical Reports, Series No. 10, Medical Uses of Ca^{47}. Vienna: International Atomic Energy Agency 1962, p. 80.
— — — PAZIANOS, A., PEARSON, O. H., LAUGHLIN, J. S.: The use of calcium 47 in diagnostic studies of patients with bone lesions. Amer. J. Roentgenol. 85, 955 (1961).
CRAMER, C. F.: Quantitative studies on the absorption and excretion of calcium from Thiry-Vella intestinal loops in the dog. In: The Tranfser of Calcium and Strontium Across Biological Membranes. Ed.: R. H. WASSERMAN. New York-London: Academic Press 1963, p. 75.
CUNLIFFE, W. J., BLACK, M. M., HALL, R., JOHNSTON, I. D., HUDGSON, P., SHUSTER, S., GUDMUNDSSON, T. V., JOPLIN, G. F., WILLIAMS, E. D., WOODHOUSE, N. J. Y., GALANTE, L., MACINTYRE, I.: A calcitonin-secreting thyroid carcinoma. Lancet 1968 II, 63.
D'ABRAMO, F., LIPMANN, F.: The formation of adenosine-3'-phosphate-5'-phosphosulfate in extracts of chick embryo cartilage and its conversion into chondroitin sulfate. Biochem. biophys. Acta (Amst.) 25, 211 (1957).
DALE, N. E., KELLERMAN, G. M.: The binding of calcium by the plasma proteins in hyperparathyroidism. Clin. Sci. 32, 433 (1967).
DANISHEFSKY, I., EIBER, H. B.: Studies on the metabolism of heparin. Arch. Biochem. 85, 53 (1959).
DAVIDSON, E. A., SMALL, W.: Metabolism in vivo of connective-tissue mucopolysaccharides. III. Chondroitin sulfate and keratosulfate of cartilage. Biochim. biophys. Acta (Amst.) 69, 459 (1963).
DAVIGNON, J., SIMMONDS, W. J., AHRENS, E. H., JR.: Usefulness of chromic oxide as an internal standard for balance studies in formula-fed patients and for assessment of colonic function. J. clin. Invest. 47, 127 (1968).
DELLA ROSA, R. J., GOLDMAN, M., ANDERSEN, A. C., MAYS, C. W., STOVER, B. J.: Absorption and retention of ingested strontium and calcium in beagles as a function of age. Nature 205, 197 (1965).
DE SOMER, L., COENEGRACHT, J., DORLEYN, M.: Disorders of calcium metabolism investigated with strontium 85. Acta med. scand. 175, 653 (1964).

DEYL, Z., ROSMUS, J., BUMP, S.: Studies on the structure of collagen. II. The nature of the N- and C-terminals in enzyme-treated and untreated collagen. Biochim. biophys. Acta (Amst.) 140, 515 (1967).

DORFMAN, A.: The biosynthesis of acid mucopolysaccharides. In: Structure and Function of Connective and Skeletal Tissue. Eds.: S. FITTON JACKSON, R. D. HARKNESS, S. M. PARTRIDGE, and G. TRISTRAM. London: Butterworths 1965, p. 297.

DYMLING, J. F.: Calcium kinetics in oesteopenia and parathyroid disease. Acta med. scand. 175, Suppl. 408 (1964).

EANES, E. D., POSNER, A. S.: Kinetics and mechanism of conversion of non-crystalline calcium phosphate to crystalline hydroxyapatite. Trans. N. Y. Acad. Sci. 28, 233 (1965).

EFRON, M. L., BIXBY, E. M., HOCKADAY, T. D. R., SMITH, L. H., JR., MESHORER, E.: Hydroxyprolinemia. III. The origin of free hydroxyproline in hydroxyprolinemia. Collagen turnover. Evidence for a biosynthetic pathway in man. Biochim. biophys. Acta (Amst.) 165, 238 (1968).

ENGSTROM, A.: Ultrastructure of bone mineral. In: Bone as a Tissue. Eds.: K. RODAHL, J. T. NICHOLSON, and E. M. BROWN, JR. New York: McGraw-Hill Book Company 1960, p. 251.

ESTEP, H. L., GARDNER, C. T., JR., TAYLOR, J. P., MINOTT, A., TUCKER, H. ST. GEORGE, JR.: Phosphate excretion patterns following intravenous injections of ethylenediaminetetraacetate (EDTA). J. clin. Endocr. 25, 1385 (1965).

FERRI, G., CASTELLANI, A. A., ZAMBOTTI, V.: Presenza di acido sialico nella cartilagine metafisaria. R. C. Ist. Lombardo 93, 214 (1959).

FITTON JACKSON, S.: Macromolecular order in the ground substance. In: Structure and Function of Connective and Skeletal Tissue. Eds.: S. FITTON JACKSON, R. D. HARKNESS, S. M. PARTRIDGE, and G. R. TRISTRAM. London: Butterworths 1965, p. 156.

FLEISCH, H., and BISAZ, S.: Mechanism of calcification: inhibitory role of pyrophosphate. Nature 195, 911 (1962).

— — Role of collagen, pyrophosphate and pyrophosphatase in calcification. In: Bone and Tooth. Ed.: H. J. J. BLACKWOOD. Oxford: Pergamon Press 1964, p. 249.

— — On the role of condensed phosphates in the regulation of calcification. In: Structure and Function of Connective and Skeletal Tissue. Eds.: S. FITTON JACKSON, R. D. HARKNESS, S. M. PARTRIDGE, and G. R. TRISTRAM. London: Butterworths 1965, p. 347.

— —, CARE, A. D.: Effect of orthophosphate on urinary pyrophosphate excretion and the prevention of urolithiasis. Lancet 1964 I, 1065.

—, MAERKI, J., RUSSELL, R. G. G.: Effect of pyrophosphate on dissolution of hydroxyapatite and its possible importance in calcium homeostasis. Proc. Soc. exp. Biol. (N. Y.) 122, 317 (1966 a).

—, NEUMAN, W. F.: Mechanism of calcification: role of collagen, polyphosphates, and phosphatase. Amer. J. Physiol. 200, 1296 (1961).

—, RUSSELL, R. G. G., STRAUMANN, F.: Effect of pyrophosphate on hydroxyapatite and its implications in calcium homeostasis. Nature 212, 901 (1966 b).

FRANZBLAU, C., SEIFTER, S., GALLOP, P. M.: The nondialysable fraction obtained from ichtyocol digested with collagenase. Biopolymers 2, 185 (1964).

FRIIS, T., HAHNEMANN, S., WEEKE, E.: Serum calcium and serum phosphorus in uraemia during administration of sodium phytate and aluminium hydroxide. Acta med. scand. 183, 497 (1968).

FURTH, J.: Hormones and neoplasia. In: Cancer and Aging. Eds.: A. ENGEL and T. LARSSON. Stockholm: Nordiska Bokhandelns Förlag 1968, p. 131.

GESCHWIND, I. I.: Hormonal control of calcium, phosphorus, iodine, iron, sulfur, and magnesium metabolism. In: Mineral Metabolism, v. 1-B. Eds.: C. L. COMAR and F. BRONNER. New York-London: Academic Press 1961, p. 387.

GLIMCHER, M. J.: Specificity of the molecular structure of organic matrices in mineralization. In: Calcification in Biological Systems. Ed.: R. F. SOGNNAES. Washington: Amer. Ass. Advanc. Sci. 1960, p. 421.

—, ANDRIKIDES, A., KOSSIVA, D.: Studies on the mechanism of calcification. I. The alteration of amino acid side chain groups of collagen and its effect on in vitro calcification. In:

Structure and Function of Connective and Skeletal Tissue. Eds.: S. FITTON JACKSON, R. D. HARKNESS, S. M. PARTRIDGE, and G. R. TRISTRAM. London: Butterworths 1965, p. 342.

GOMORI, G.: A modification of colorimetric phosphorus determination for use with photo-electric colorimeter. J. Lab. clin. Med. 27, 955 (1942).

GORDAN, G. S.: Hormonal effects of nonendocrine tumours with special reference to the hypercalcaemia of breast cancer. In: Current Concepts in Breast Cancer. Ed.: A. SEGALOFF. Baltimore: Williams & Wilkins 1967, p. 132.

—, CANTINO, T. J., ERHARDT, L., HANSEN, J., LUBICH, W.: Osteolytic sterol in human breast cancer. Science 151, 1226 (1966).

GRASSMANN, W., HANNIG, K., NORDWIG, A.: Über die apolaren Bereiche des Kollagenmoleküles. Z. Physiol. Chem. 333, 154 (1963).

HAAGENSEN, C. D., COOLEY, E.: Treatment of early mammary carcinoma. A cooperative international study. Ann. Surg. 157, 157 (1963).

HARRIS, E. D., JR., MUNOZ, A. J., KRANE, S. M.: Excretion of collagen-like fragments in the urine of patients with Paget's disease of bone. J. clin. Invest. (Abstr.) 46, 1066 (1967).

HART, H., SPENCER, H.: Rate of initial entry of Ca^{47} and Sr^{85} from the intestine into the vascular space. Proc. Soc. exp. Biol. (N. Y.) 126, 365 (1967).

HASSID, W. Z.: Biosynthesis of complex saccharides. In: Metabolic Pathways, v. 1. Ed.: D. M. GREENBERG. New York-London: Academic Press 1967, p. 307.

HAZARD, J. B., HAWK, W. A., CRILE, G., JR.: Medullary (solid) carcinoma of thyroid: clinicopathological entity. J. clin. Endocr. 19, 152 (1959).

HEANEY, R. P.: Evaluation and interpretation of calcium-kinetic data in man. Clin. Orthop. 31, 153 (1964).

—, BAUER, G. C. H., BRONNER, F., DYMLING, J. F., LAFFERTY, F. W., NORDIN, B. E. C., RICH, C.: A normal reference standard for radiocalcium turnover and excretion in humans. J. Lab. clin. Med. 64, 21 (1964).

—, WHEDON, G. D.: Radiocalcium studies of bone formation rate in human metabolic bone disease. J. clin. Endocr. 18, 1246 (1958).

HERRMAN, J. B., KIRSTEN, E., KRAKAUER, J. S.: Hypercalcemic syndrome associated with androgenic and estrogenic therapy. J. clin. Endocr. 9, 1 (1949).

HIRSCH, P. F., VOELKEL, E. F., MUNSON, P. L.: Thyrocalcitonin: hypocalcemic, hypophosphatemic principle of the thyroid gland. Science 146, 412 (1964).

HORTON, J., OLSON, K. B.: Hypercalcaemia associated with cancer of the breast and other organs. In: Bone and Tooth. Ed.: H. J. J. BLACKWOOD. Oxford-London-New York-Paris: Pergamon Press 1964, p. 207.

IRVING, J. T.: Dynamics and function of phosphorus. In: Mineral Metabolism, v. 2-A. Eds.: C. L. COMAR and F. BRONNER. New York-London: Academic Press 1964, p. 249.

JAFFE, H. L.: Tumors and Tumorous Conditions of the Bones and Joints. Philadelphia: Lea and Febiger 1958.

JASIN, H. E., FINK, C. W., WIZE, W., ZIFF, M.: Relationship between urinary hydroxyproline and growth. J. clin. Invest. 41, 1928 (1962).

JOHNSTON, C. C., JR., DEISS, W. P., JR., FRENCH, R. S.: Effect of changes in parathyroid status and calcium equilibrium on bone matrix metabolism. Proc. Soc. exp. Biol. (N. Y.) 118, 551 (1965).

JOWSEY, J., GERSHON-COHEN, J.: Clinical and experimental osteoporosis. In: Bone and Tooth. Ed.: H. J. J. BLACKWOOD. Oxford-London-New York-Paris: Pergamon Press 1964, p. 35.

KALLFELZ, F. A., TAYLOR, A. N., WASSERMAN, R. H.: Vitamin D-induced calcium binding factor in rat intestinal mucosa. Proc. Soc. exp. Biol. (N. Y.) 125, 54 (1967).

KAPLAN, D., McKUSICK, V., TREBACH, S., LAZARUS, R.: Keratosulfate-chondroitin sulfate peptide from normal urine and from urine of patients with Morquio syndrome (Mucopolysaccharidosis IV). J. Lab. clin. Med. 71, 48 (1968).

KATZ, F. H.: Effects of oestradiol and oestriol on the disposition of injected radioactive proline, hydroxyproline and tyrosine in man. Acta Endocr. 58, 664 (1968).

—, KAPPAS, A.: Influence of estradiol and estriol on urinary excretion of hydroxyproline in man. J. Lab. clin. Med. 71, 65 (1968).

KENNEDY, B. J., NATHANSON, I. I., TIBBETS, D. M., AUB, J. C.: Biochemical alterations during steroid hormone therapy for advanced breast cancer. Amer. J. Med. 19, 337 (1955).

KENNEDY, B. J., TIBBETS, D. M., NATHANSON, I. I., AUB, J. C.: Hypercalcaemia, a complication of hormone therapy of advanced breast cancer. Cancer Res. 13, 445 (1953).

KING, E. J., WOOTTON, I. D. P.: Micro-Analysis in Medical Biochemistry, 3rd ed. London: J. and A. Churchill 1956, p. 81.

KIVIRIKKO, K. I., PROCKOP, D. J.: Hydroxylation of proline in synthetic polypeptides with purified protocollagen hydroxylase. J. biol. Chem. 242, 4007 (1967).

KLEEMAN, C. R., ROCKNEY, R. E., MAXWELL, M. H.: The effect of parathyroid extract (PTE) on the renal clearance of diffusible calcium. J. clin. Invest. (Abstr.) 37, 907 (1958).

KLEIN, D. C., MORII, H., TALMAGE, R. V.: Effect of thyrocalcitonin, administered during peritoneal lavage, on removal of bone salts and their radioisotopes. Proc. Soc. exp. Biol. (N. Y.) 124, 627 (1967).

—, TALMAGE, R. V.: Thyrocalcitonin suppression of hydroxyproline release from bone. Proc. exp. Biol. (N. Y.) 127, 95 (1968).

KOHLER, H. F., PECHET, M.: The inhibition of bone resorption by thyrocalcitonin. J. clin. Invest. (Abstr.) 45, 1033 (1966).

KRAWITT, E. L.: Effect of thyrocalcitonin on duodenal calcium transport. Proc. Soc. exp. Biol. (N. Y.) 125, 1084 (1967).

LAFFERTY, F. W., SPENCER, G. E., PEARSON, O. H.: Effects of androgens, estrogens and high calcium intakes on bone formation and resorption in osteoporosis. Amer. J. Med. 36, 514 (1964).

LAITINEN, O.: The metabolism of collagen and its hormonal control in the rat. Acta Endocr. Suppl. 120 (1967).

LASSITER, W. E., GOTTSCHALK, C. W., MYLLE, M.: Micropuncture study of renal tubular reabsorption of calcium in normal rodents. Amer. J. Physiol. 204, 771 (1963).

LASZLO, D., SCHULMAN, C. A., BELLIN, S., GOTTESMAN, F. D., SCHILLING, A.: Mineral and protein metabolism in osteolytic metastases. J. Amer. med. Ass. 148, 1027 (1952).

LAX, L. C., SIDLOFSKY, S., WRENSHALL, G. A.: Compartmental contents and simultaneous transfer rates of phosphorus in the rat. J. Physiol. 132, 1 (1956).

LAZOR, M. Z., ROSENBERG, L. E.: Mechanism of adrenal-steroid reversal of hypercalcemia in multiple myeloma. New Engl. J. Med. 270, 749 (1964).

LERCH, P., VUILLEUMIER, C.: Physico-chemical methods for the identification of microcrystalline basic calcium phosphates prepared in vitro. In: Calcified Tissues 1965. Eds.: H. FLEISCH, H. J. J. BLACKWOOD, and M. OWEN. Berlin-Heidelberg: Springer 1966, p. 132.

LEWALLEN, C. G., BERMAN, M., RALL, J. E.: Studies of iodoalbumin metabolism. I. A mathematical approach to the kinetics. J. clin. Invest 38, 66 (1959).

LEWISON, E. F.: Castration in the treatment of advanced breast cancer. Cancer 18, 1558 (1965).

LINDSTEDT, S., PROCKOP, D. J.: Isotopic studies on urinary hydroxyproline as evidence for rapidly catabolized forms of collagen in the young rat. J. biol. Chem. 236, 1399 (1961).

LLOYD, A. C., EMBERY, G., WUSTEMAN, F. S., LARGE, P. J. DODGSON, K. S.: The catabolism of sulphated glycosaminoglycans. In: Structure and Function of Connective and Skeletal Tissue. Eds.: S. FITTON JACKSON, R. D. HARKNESS, S. M. PARTRIDGE, and G. R. TRISTRAM. London: Butterworths 1965, p. 459.

LLOYD, E.: Relative binding of strontium and calcium in protein and non-protein fractions of serum in the rabbit. Nature 217, 355 (1968).

LOKEN, H. F., GORDAN, G. S.: Renal mechanisms in the production of hypercalcaemia in hyperparathyroidism and breast cancer. J. clin. Invest. (Abstr.) 38, 1021 (1959).

LOUGH, S. A., HAMADA, G. H., COMAR, C. L.: Secretion of dietary strontium 90 and calcium in human milk. Proc. Soc. exp. Biol. (N. Y.) 104, 194 (1960).

LUTWAK, L., BURTON, B. T.: Fecal dye markers in metabolic balance studies. The use of brilliant blue and methylcellulose for accurate separation of stool periods. Amer. J. clin. Nutr. 14, 109 (1964).

MACINTYRE, J., FOSTER, G. V., CUMAR, M. A.: Calcitonin. Proc. roy. Soc. Med. 57, 865 (1964).

MANNER, G., KRETSINGER, R. H., GOULD, B. S., RICH, A.: The polyribosomal synthesis of collagen. Biochim. biophys. Acta (Amst.) 134, 411 (1967).

MARINO, A. A., BECKER, R. O.: Evidence for direct physical bonding between the collagen fibres and apatite crystals in bone. Nature 213, 697 (1967).

MARSHALL, J. H.: Theory of alkaline earth metabolism. The power function makes possible a simple but comprehensive model of skeletal system. J. theor. Biol. 6, 386 (1964).

MATHEWS, M. B.: Molecular evolution of connective tissue. A comparative study of acid mucopolysaccharide-protein complexes. In: Structure and Function of Connective and Skeletal Tissue. Eds.: S. FITTON JACKSON, R. D. HARKNESS, S. M. PARTRIDGE, and G. R. TRISTRAM. London: Butterworths 1965, p. 181.

—, LOSAITYTE, I.: Sodium chondroitin sulfate-protein complexes of cartilage. I. Molecular weight and shape. Arch. Biochem. Biophys. 74, 158 (1958).

MATHISON, G. C.: The estimation of phosphorus in urine. Biochem. J. 4, 233 (1909).

McCREADY, V. R., COTTRALL, M. F., FIELD, E. O., FRENCH, R. J., TROTT, N. G.: The detection of metastases in the skeleton using radioactive isotopes. Brit. J. Radiol. 39, 791 (1966).

McLEAN, F. C., BUDY, A. M.: Radiation, Isotopes, and Bone. New York-London: Academic Press 1964.

—, HASTINGS, A. B.: The state of calcium in the fluids of the body. I. The conditions affecting the ionization of calcium. J. biol. Chem. 108, 285 (1935).

McPHERSON, G. D.: Stable calcium isotopes as tracers in studies of mineral metabolism. Acta orthop. scand. Suppl. 78 (1965).

MEEMA, H. E., BUNKER, M. L., MEEMA, S.: Loss of compact bone due to menopause. Obstet. and Gynec. 26, 333 (1965).

—, MEEMA, S.: Prevention of postmenopausal osteoporosis by hormone treatment of the menopause. Canad. med. Ass. J. 99, 248 (1968).

MEILMAN, E., URIVETZKY, M. M., RAPOPORT, C. M.: Urinary hydroxyproline peptides. J. clin. Invest. 42, 40 (1963).

MEYER, J. S., ABDEL-BARI, W.: Granules and thyrocalcitonin-like activity in medullary carcinoma of the thyroid gland. New Engl. J. Med. 278, 530 (1968).

MEYER, K., ANDERSON, B., SENO, N., HOFFMAN, P.: Peptide complexes of chondroitin sulphates and keratosulphates. In: Structure and Function of Connective and Skeletal Tissue. Eds.: S. FITTON JACKSON, R. D. HARKNESS, S. M. PARTRIDGE, and G. R. TRISTRAM. London: Butterworths 1965, p. 164.

MILHAUD, G., MOUKHTAR, M. S.: Antagonistic and synergistic actions of thyrocalcitonin and parathyroid hormone on the levels of calcium and phosphate in the rat. Nature 211, 1186 (1966 a).

— — Thyrocalcitonin: Effects on calcium kinetics in the rat. Proc. Soc. exp. Biol. (N. Y.) 123, 207 (1966 b).

MILLER, E. J., MARTIN, G. R., PIEZ, K. A., POWERS, M. J.: Characterization of chick bone collagen and compositional changes associated with maturation. J. biol. Chem. 242, 5481 (1967).

MUIRHEAD, W.: Hormonal treatment of hypercalcemia caused by bone metastases. Canad. med. Ass. J. 97, 569 (1967).

MUNSON, P. L.: Thyrocalcitonin. Ann. Intern. Med. 64, 1353 (1966).

MYERS, W. P. L.: Hypercalcemia in neoplastic disease. Arch. Surg. 80, 308 (1960).

—, GREENBERG, E. J., ROTHSCHILD, E. O., MERLINO, M., WEBER, D. A., COREY, K. R.: $^{47}Ca/^{85}Sr$ studies of the mechanism of the hypercalcemia of cancer. J. clin. Invest. (Abstr.) 45, 1034 (1966).

—, ROTHSCHILD, E. O., CARNEY, V., KAPLAN, N., GREENBERG, E. J., DIMICH, A., WEBER, D.: Tumor-induced hypercalcemia: radiocalcium and bone culture studies. Calc. Tiss. Res. 2, Suppl., 63 (1968).

NEER, R., BERMAN, M., FISHER, L., ROSENBERG, L. E.: Multicompartmental analysis of calcium kinetics in normal adult males. J. clin. Invest. 46, 1364 (1967).

NEHER, R., RINIKER, B., MAIER, R., BYFIELD, P. G. H., GUDMUNDSSON, T. V., MacINTYRE, I.: Human calcitonin. Nature 220, 984 (1968).

NEUMAN, R. E., LOGAN, M. A.: The determination of collagen and elastin in tissues. J. biol. Chem. 186, 549 (1950).

NISSEN-MEYER, R., SANNER, T.: The excretion of oestrone, pregnanediol and pregnanetriol in breast cancer patients. I. Excretion after spontaneous menopause. Acta Endocr. **44**, 325 (1963 a).

— — The excretion of oestrone, pregnanediol and pregnanetriol in breast cancer patients. II. Effect of ovariectomy, ovarian irradiation and corticosteroids. Acta Endocr. **44**, 334 (1963 b).

NORDIN, B. E .C.: Osteoporosis and calcium deficiency. In: Bone as a Tissue. Eds.: K. RODAHL, J. T. NICHOLSON, and E. M. BROWN, JR.: New York: McGraw-Hill Book Company 1960, p. 46.

—, FRASER, R.: Assessment of urinary phosphate excretion. Lancet 1960 I, 947.

O'RIORDAN, J. L. H.: Thyrocalcitonin. Ann. intern. Med. **67**, 903 (1967).

OWEN, M.: Cell population kinetics of an osteogenic tissue. I. J. cell. Biol. **19**, 19 (1963).

PAK, C. Y. C., BARTTER, F. C.: Ionic interaction with bone mineral. I. Evidence for an isoionic calcium exchange with hydroxyapatite. Biochim. biophys. Acta (Amst.) **141**, 401 (1967 a).

— — Ionic interaction with bone mineral. II. The control of Ca^{2+} and PO_4^{3-} exchange by univalent cation- Ca^{2+} substitution at the hydroxyapatite crystal surface. Biochim. biophys. Acta (Amst.) **141**, 410 (1967 b).

PARTRIDGE, S. M., WHITING, A. H., DAVIS, H. F.: The presence of aggregates containing non-covalently linked protein in preparations of the chondroitin sulphate-protein complex from bovine cartilage. In: Structure and Function of Connective and Skeletal Tissue. Eds.: S. FITTON JACKSON, R. D. HARKNESS, S. M. PARTRIDGE, and G. R. TRISTRAM. London: Butterworths 1965, p. 160.

PEARSON, J. D.: Use of Cr^{51}-labelled haemoglobin and Sc^{47} as inert faecal markers. Int. J. appl. Radiat. **17**, 13 (1966).

PELLEGRINO, E. D., BILTZ, R. M.: Bone carbonate and the Ca to P molar ratio. Nature **219**, 1261 (1968).

PERSSON, B. H., RISHOLM, L.: Oophorectomy and cortisone treatment as a method of eliminating oestrogen production in patients with breast cancer. Acta Endocr. **47**, 15 (1964).

—, WEST, C. D., HOLLANDER, V. P., TREVES, N. E.: Evaluation of endocrine therapy for advanced breast cancer. J. Amer. med. Ass. **154**, 234 (1954).

PETERS, J. P., VAN SLYKE, D. D.: Quantitative Clinical Chemistry, Methods, v. II. Baltimore: Williams & Wilkins 1961.

PETRUSKA, J. A., HODGE, A. J.: A subunit model for the tropocollagen macromolecule. Proc. nat. Acad. Sci. (Wash.) **51**, 871 (1964).

PHANG, J. M., FINERMAN, G. A. M., BERMAN, M., ROSENBERG, L. E.: Coordinated target organ responses to parathyroid hormone. J. clin. Invest. (Abstr.) **46**, 1104 (1967).

PIEZ, K. A.: Nonidentity of the three α chains in codfish skin collagen. J. biol. Chem. **239**, PC 4315 (1964).

PLIMPTON, C. H., GELLHORN, A.: Hypercalcemia in malignant disease without evidence of bone destruction. Amer. J. Med. **21**, 750 (1956).

POSNER, A. S.: The nature of the inorganic phase in calcified tissues. In: Calcification in Biological Systems. Ed.: R. F. SOGNNAES. Washington: Amer. Ass. Advanc. Sci. 1960, p. 373.

PRASAD, A. S., FLINK, E. B.: The determination of ultrafiltrable calcium in a variety of clinical conditions. J. Lab. clin. Med. **52**, 1 (1958).

PRINS, J. A.: Structure of non-crystalline solids. In: Physics of Non-crystalline Solids. Ed.: J. A. PRINS. New York: Interscience 1965, p. 1.

PROCKOP, D. J.: Isotopic studies on collagen degradation and the urine excretion of hydroxyproline. J. clin. Invest. **43**, 453 (1964).

—, KIVIRIKKO, K. I.: Relationship of hydroxyproline excretion in urine to collagen metabolism. Ann. intern. Med. **66**, 1243 (1967).

PROCOPÉ, B.-J.: Studies on the urinary excretion, biological effects and origin of oestrogens in post-menopausal women. Acta Endocr. **60**, Suppl., 135 (1969).

RAISZ, L. G., NIEMANN, I.: Early effects of parathyroid hormone on bone in tissue culture. J. clin. Invest. (Abstr.) **45**, 1059 (1966).

RAMACHANDRAN, G. N.: Molecular structure of collagen. In: Intern. Rev. Connective Tissue Res., v. 1. Ed.: D. A. HALL. New York: Academic Press 1963, p. 127.

RANDALL, R. E., JR., LIRENMAN, D. S.: Hypocalcemia and hypophosphatemia accompanying osteoblastic metastases. J. clin. Endocr. (letter) 24, 1331 (1964).

RASMUSSEN, H., ANAST, C., ARNAUD, C.: Thyrocalcitonin, EGTA, and urinary electrolyte excretion. J. clin. Invest. 46, 746 (1967).

—, ARNAUD, C., HAWKER, C.: Actinomycin D and the response to parathyroid hormone. Science 144, 1019 (1964).

RAWSON, A. J., SUNDERMAN, F. W.: Studies in serum electrolytes. XV. The calcium binding property of serum proteins (multiple myeloma, lymphogranuloma venereum, and sarcoidosis). J. clin. Invest. 27, 82 (1948).

RAYNAUD, C., KELLERSHOHN, C.: Mesure des compartiments rapidement échangeables, des taux d'échange et de transfert du magnésium à l'aide du ^{28}Mg chez l'adulte normal et pathologique. Nucl. Med. 5, 211 (1966).

REIFENSTEIN, E. C., JR., ALBRIGHT, F., WELLS, S. L.: The accumulation, interpretation, and presentation of data pertaining to metabolic balances, notably those of calcium, phosphorus, and nitrogen. J. clin. Endocr. 5, 367 (1945), and erratum 6, 232 (1946).

RICH, C., ENSINCK, J., FELLOWS, H.: The use of continuous infusions of calcium^{45} and strontium^{85} to study skeletal function. J. clin. Endocr. 21, 611 (1961).

RINIKER, B., NEHER, R., MAIER, R., KAHNT, F. W., BYFIELD, P. G. H., GUDMUNDSSON, T. V., GALANTE, L., MacINTYRE, I.: Menschliches Calcitonin. I. Isolierung und Charakterisierung. Helv. chim. Acta 51, 1738 (1968).

RODÉN, L., SMITH, R.: Structure of the neutral trisaccharide of the chondroitin 4-sulfate-protein linkage region. J. biol. Chem. 241, 5949 (1966).

ROSE, G. A.: Determination of the ionised and ultrafilterable calcium of normal human plasma. Clin. chim. Acta 2, 227 (1957).

— Immobilization osteoporosis; a study of the extent, severity, and treatment with bendrofluazide. Brit. J. Surg. 53, 769 (1966).

ROSENBLOOM, J., BHATNAGAR, R. S., PROCKOP, D. J.: Hydroxylation of proline after the release of proline-rich polypeptides from ribosomal complexes during uninhibited collagen synthesis. Biochim. biophys. Acta (Amst.) 149, 259 (1967).

ROSMUS, J., DEYL, Z., DRAKE, M. P.: Studies on the structure of collagen. I. The sequence analysis of peptides released by pronase. Biochim. biophys. Acta (Amst.) 140, 507 (1967).

SAMACHSON, J.: The gastrointestinal clearance of strontium-85 and calcium-45 in man. Radiat. Res. 27, 64 (1966).

— Mechanism for the exchange of the calcium in bone mineral. Nature 216, 193 (1967).

—, KABAKOW, B., SPENCER, H.: Comparative passage of Sr^{85} and Ca^{45} from plasma into body fluids in man. Proc. Soc. exp. (N. Y.) 103, 570 (1960).

—, VANKINSCOTT, V., SPENCER, H.: Secretion of Sr^{85} and Ca^{47} in human saliva. Proc. Soc. exp. Biol. (N. Y.) 118, 747 (1965).

SEIFERT, G., SEEMANN, N.: Paraneoplastisches Hypercalcaemie-Syndrom bei Ovarialkarzinom. Dtsch. med. Wschr. 92, 1104 (1967).

SEIFTER, S., FRANZBLAU, C., HARPER, E., GALLOP, P. M.: Special aspects of the primary structure of collagen. In: Structure and Function of Connective and Skeletal Tissue. Eds.: S. FITTON JACKSON, R. D. HARKNESS, S. M. PARTRIDGE, and G. R. TRISTRAM. London: Butterworths 1965, p. 21.

SENO, N., MEYER, K., ANDERSON, B., HOFFMAN, P.: Variations in keratosulfates. J. biol. Chem. 240, 1005 (1965).

SHERWOOD, L. M., MAYER, G. P., RAMBERG, C. F., JR., KRONFELD, D. S., POTTS, J. T., JR., AURBACH, G. D.: The relative importance of calcium and phosphate in the secretion of parathyroid hormone. J. clin. Invest. (Abstr.) 45, 1072 (1966).

—, O'RIORDAN, J. L. H., AURBACH, G. D., POTTS, J. T., JR.: Production of parathyroid hormones by non-parathyroid tumors. J. clin. Endocr. 27, 140 (1967).

SILBERT, J. E.: Biosynthesis of heparin. III. Formation of a sulfated glycosaminoglycan with a microsomal preparation from mast cell tumors. J. biol. Chem. 242, 5146 (1967).

SIMMONS, D. J.: Collagen formation and endochondral ossification in estrogen treated mice. Proc. Soc. exp. Biol. (N. Y.) 121, 1165 (1966).

SKLAROFF, D. M., CHARKES, N. D.: The value of strontium 85 bone scanning in radiation therapy. Amer. J. Roentgenol. 99, 415 (1967 a).
— — The early detection of bone metastasis in patients with stage II carcinoma of the breast at time of radical surgery. J. nucl. Med. (Abstr.) 8, 272 (1967 b).
SLATOPOLSKY, E., GRADOWSKA, L., KASHEMSANT, C., KELTNER, R., MANLEY, C., BRICKER, N. S.: The control of phosphate excretion in uremia. J. clin. Invest. 45, 672 (1966).
SMARSZ, C.: Prosta metoda ultrasączenia jako wstępna czynność rozdzielania frakcji wapnia w płynach biologicznych. (A simple method of ultrafiltration for initial separation of calcium fractions in biological fluids.) Pol. Arch. Med. wewnęt. 38, 767 (1967).
— Serum protein pattern and serum calcium, magnesium and inorganic phosphate fractions and their dissociation constants. Pol. Arch. Med. wewnęt. (in the press).
—, ADAMSKI, A.: Serum protein pattern and serum calcium fractions in various diseases. (In Polish.) Pol. Arch. Med. wewnęt. 38, 773 (1967).
SMITH, J. W.: Molecular pattern in native collagen. Nature 219, 157 (1968).
SNEDECOR, G. W.: Statistical Methods Applied to Experiments in Agriculture and Biology, 5th ed. Ames (Iowa): Iowa State University Press 1956.
SOLIMAN, H. A., ROBINSON, C. J. FOSTER, G. V., MACINTYRE, I.: Mode of action of calcitonin. In: Calcified Tissues 1965. Eds.: H. FLEISCH, H. J. J. BLACKWOOD, and M. OWEN. Berlin-Heidelberg-New York: Springer 1966, p. 242.
SOLOMON, A. K.: Compartmental methods of kinetic analysis. In: Mineral Metabolism, v. 1-A. Eds.: C. L. COMAR and F. BRONNER. New York-London: Academic Press 1960, p. 119.
SPENCER, H., LEWIN, I., SAMACHSON, J.: Influence of dietary calcium intake on the calcium/strontium discrimination ratio in man. Radiat. Res. (Abstr.) 27, Fc3 (1966).
SPENCER, R., HERBERT, R., RISH, M. W., LITTLE, W. A.: Bone scanning with ^{85}Sr, ^{87m}Sr and ^{18}F; physical and radiopharmaceutical considerations and clinical experience in 50 cases. Brit. J. Radiol. 40, 641 (1967).
STANLEY, M. M., CHENG, S. H.: Excretion from the gut and gastrointestinal exchange studied by means of the inert indicator method. Amer. J. dig. Dis. 2, 628 (1957).
STERN, B. D., GLIMCHER, M. J., MECHANIC, G. L., GOLDHABER, P.: Studies of collagen degradation during bone resorption in tissue culture. Proc. Soc. exp. Biol. (N. Y.) 119, 557 (1965).
STEVEN, F. S.: Multiple-stage depolymerisation of collagen fibrils. Biochim. biophys. Acta (Amst.) 130, 202 (1966).
STROTT, C. A., NUGENT, C. A.: Laboratory tests in the diagnosis of hyperparathyroidism in hypercalcemic patients. Ann. intern. Med. 68, 188 (1968).
SZYMENDERA, J.: Methods of chemical assay of calcium: In: Technical Reports Series No. 32, Medical Uses of Ca^{47}: Second Panel Report. Vienna: International Atomic Energy Agency 1964, p. 163.
—, LEWINSKI, T., NOWOSIELSKI, J., RADOM, S., TOLWINSKI, J.: Determination of the extracellular water volume by means of ^{35}S-radiosulphate. Bull. Acad. pol. Sci. Cl. VI. 14, 135 (1966).
—, MADAJEWICZ, S.: Calcium metabolism after castration. Lancet 1967 II, 1091.
— — Comparative ultrafiltrability of calcium and strontium in human plasma. Nature 217, 968 (1968).
— — Tests of renal handling of inorganic phosphate: Comparison of data based on total and diffusible inorganic plasma phosphate concentration. (In press.)
—, STANKOWSKA, A., TOLWINSKI, J., ZULAWSKI, M., NOWOSIELSKI, J., JASINSKI, W. K.: A critical analysis of calcium kinetics in metastatic cancer. Nucl. Med. 6, 273 (1967 a).
—, TOLWINSKI, J., JASINSKI, W. K.: Calcium kinetics in malignancy without skeletal involvement. Nucl. Med. 6, 265 (1967 b).
TASHJIAN, A. H., LEVINE, L., MUNSON, P. L.: Immunochemical identification of parathyroid hormone in non-parathyroid neoplasms associated with hypercalcaemia. J. exp. Med. 119, 467 (1964).
TAUSSKY, H. H., BRAHEN, L.: Creatinine and creatine in urine and serum. In: Standard Methods of Clinical Chemistry, v. 3. Ed.: D. SELIGSON. New York-London: Academic Press 1961, p. 99.
TAYLOR, A. N., WASSERMAN, R. H.: A vitamin D$_3$-dependent factor influencing calcium binding by homogenates of chick intestinal mucosa. Nature 205, 248 (1965).

TERMINE, J. D., POSNER, A. S.: Infrared analysis of rat bone: age dependency of amorphous and crystalline mineral fractions. Science 153, 1523 (1966).
— — Amorphous/crystalline interrelationship in bone mineral. Calc. Tiss. Res. 1, 8 (1967).
—, WUTHIER, R. E., POSNER, A. S.: Amorphous-crystalline mineral changes during endochondral and periosteal bone formation. Proc. Soc. exp. Biol. (N. Y.) 125, 4 (1967).
THOMAS, A. N., LOKEN, H. F., GORDAN, G. S., GOLDMAN, L.: Hypercalcemia of metastatic breast cancer. Surg. Forum 11, 70 (1960).
TRANSBØL, I., HAHNEMANN, S., HORNUM, I.: The tubular reabsorption of calcium in primary hyperparathyroidism and in non-parathyroid hypercalcemia. Acta med. scand. 184, 33 (1968).
VAES, G.: Acid hydrolases, lysosomes and bone resorption induced by parathyroid hormone. In: Calcified Tissues 1965. Eds.: H. FLEISCH, H. J. J. BLACKWOOD, and M. OWEN. Berlin-Heidelberg: Springer 1966, p. 56.
WALLACH, S., HENNEMAN, P. H.: Prolonged estrogen therapy in postmenopausal women. J. Amer. med. Ass. 171, 1637 (1959).
WALSER, M.: Protein-binding of inorganic phosphate in plasma of normal subjects and patients with renal disease. J. clin. Invest. 39, 501 (1960).
— Ion Association. VI. Interactions between calcium, magnesium, inorganic phosphate, citrate and protein in normal human plasma. J. clin. Invest. 40, 723 (1961).
— The separate effects of hyperparathyroidism, hypercalcemia of malignancy, renal failure, and acidosis on the state of calcium, phosphate, and other ions in plasma. J. clin. Invest. 41, 1454 (1962).
WASE, A. W., SOLEWSKI, J., RICKES, E., SEIDENBERG, J.: Action of thyrocalcitonin on bone. Nature 214, 388 (1967).
WASSERMAN, R. H.: Metabolic basis of calcium and strontium discrimination: studies with surviving intestinal segments. Proc. Soc. exp. Biol. (N. Y.) 104, 92 (1960).
—, LENGEMANN, F. W., COMAR, C. L.: Comparative metabolism of calcium and strontium in lactation. J. Dairy Sci. 41, 812 (1958).
—, TAYLOR, A. N.: Vitamin D_3 inhibition of radiocalcium binding by chick intestinal homogenates. Nature 198, 30 (1963).
WATSON, J. D.: Involvement of RNA in the synthesis of proteins. The ordered interaction of three classes of RNA controls the assembly of amino acids into proteins. Science 140, 17 (1963).
WEISS, J. B., STEVEN, F. S.: Urinary peptides derived from the cross-linked regions of connective tissue proteins. Nature 217, 661 (1968).
WHARTON, B. A., HOWELLS, G. R., McCANCE, R. A.: Hydroxyproline indices. Nature 215, 968 (1967).
WHITBY, L. G., LANG, D.: Experience with the chromic oxide method of fecal marking in metabolic balance investigations on humans. J. clin. Invest. 39, 854 (1960).
WIDDOWSON, E. M., DICKERSON, J. W. T.: Chemical composition of the body. In: Mineral Metabolism, v. II-A. Eds.: C. L. COMAR and F. BRONNER. New York-London: Academic Press 1964, p. 1.
WILLIAMS, E. D., BROWN, C. L., DONIACH, I.: Pathological and clinical findings in series of 67 cases of medullary carcinoma of thyroid. J. clin. Path. 19, 103 (1966).
WOODARD, H. Q.: Changes in blood chemistry associated with carcinoma metastatic to bone. Cancer 6, 1219 (1953).
WOOLNER, L. B., BEAHRS, O. H., BLACK, B. M., McCONAHEY, W. M., KEATING, F. R., JR.: Classification and prognosis of thyroid carcinoma; a study of 885 cases observed in a thirty year period. Amer. J. Surg. 102, 354 (1961).
WORRALL, J., STEVEN, F. S.: The depolymerising action of pepsin on collagen. Column fractionation of the component polypeptide chains. Biochim. biophys. Acta (Amst.) 130, 184 (1966).
YOUNG, M. M., JASANI, C., SMITH, D. A., NORDIN, B. E. C.: Some effects of ethinyl oestradiol on calcium and phosphorus metabolism in osteoporosis. Clin. Sci. 34, 411 (1968).
—, NORDIN, B. E. C.: Effects of natural and artificial menopause on plasma and urinary calcium and phosphorus. Lancet 1967 II, 118.

Subject Index

Page numbers in *italics* refer to material within a table or figure

26 Tumors of the Liver. Edited by G. T. PACK and A. H. ISLAMI, New York.
    DM 56,—; US $ 15.40
27 SZYMENDERA, J., Warsaw: Bone Mineral Metabolism in Cancer. DM 32,—;
    US $ 8.80
28 MEEK, E. S., Bristol: Antitumour and Antiviral Substances of Natural Origin.
    DM 16,—; US $ 4.40

In Production

24 HAYWARD, J. L., London: Hormonal Research in Human Breast Cancer
29 Aseptic Environments and Cancer Treatment. Edited by G. MATHÉ, Villejuif
    (Symposium).
30 Advances in the Treatment of Acute (Blastic) Leukemias. Edited by G. MATHÉ,
    Villejuif (Symposium).
31 DENOIX, P., Villejuif: Treatment of Malignant Breast Tumors: Indications and
    Results
32 NELSON, R. S., Houston: Endoscopy in Gastric Cancer
33 Experimental and Clinical Effects of L-Asparaginase. Edited by E. GRUND-
    MANN, Wuppertal-Elberfeld, and H. F. OETTGEN, New York (Symposium)

In Preparation

ACKERMANN, N. B., Boston: Use of Radioisotopic Agents in the Diagnosis of
Cancer

BOIRON, M., Paris: The Viruses of the Leukemia-sarcoma Complex

CAVALIÈRE, R., A. ROSSI-FANELLI, B. MONDOVI, and G. MORICCA, Roma: Selec-
tive Heat Sensitivity of Cancer Cells

CHIAPPA, S., Milano: Endolymphatic Radiotherapy in Malignant Lymphomas

Cutane paraneoplastische Syndrome. Edited by J. J. HERZBERG, Bremen (Symposium)

GRUNDMANN, E., Wuppertal-Elberfeld: Morphologie und Cytochemie der Car-
cinogenese

IRLIN, I. S., Moskva: Mechanisms of Viral Carcinogenesis

LANGLEY, F. A., and A. C. CROMPTON, Manchester: Epithelial Abnormalities
of the Cervix Uteri

MATHÉ, G., Villejuif: L'Immunothérapie des Cancers

NEWMAN, M. K., Detroit: Neuropathies and Myopathies Associated with
Occult Malignancies

OGAWA, K., Osaka: Ultrastructural Enzyme Cytochemistry of Azo-dye Carcinogenesis

PENN, I., Denver: Malignant Lymphomas in Transplant Patients

SUGIMURA, T., Tokyo, H. ENDO, Fukuoka, and T. ONO, Tokyo: Chemistry and
Biological Action of 4-Nitroquinoline 1-oxide, a Carcinogen

WEIL, R., Lausanne: Biological and Structural Properties of Polyoma Virus
and its DNA

WILLIAMS, D. C., Caterham, Surrey: The Basis for Therapy of Hormon Sensi-
tive Tumours

WILLIAMS, D. C., Caterham, Surrey: The Biochemistry of Metastasis